www.wadsworth.com

wadsworth.com is the World Wide Web site for Wadsworth and is your direct source to dozens of online resources.

At *wadsworth.com* you can find out about supplements, demonstration software, and student resources. You can also send email to many of our authors and preview new publications and exciting new technologies.

wadsworth.com
Changing the way the world learns®

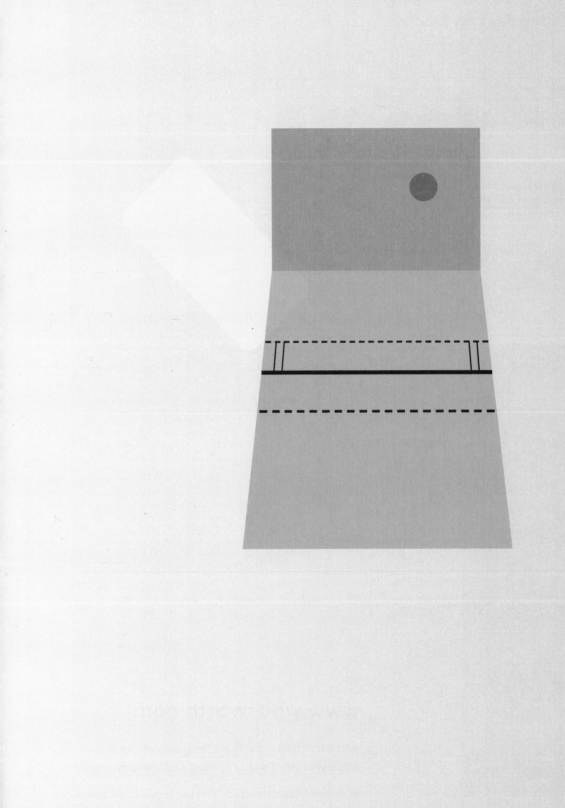

Beginning Racquetball

Fifth Edition

Cheryl Norton, Ed.D.
Metropolitan State College of Denver

James E. Bryant, Ed.D.
San Jose State University

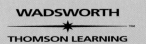

WADSWORTH

THOMSON LEARNING

Australia • Canada • Mexico • Singapore • Spain • United Kingdom • United States

WADSWORTH

™

THOMSON LEARNING

Publisher: Peter Marshall
Associate Editor: April Lemons
Assistant Editor: John Boyd
Editorial Assistant: Andrea Kesterke
Marketing Manager: Joanne Terhaar
Project Editor: Sandra Craig
Print Buyer: April Reynolds
Permissions Editor: Stephanie Keough-Hedges
Production and Composition: Ash Street Typecrafters, Inc.
Text and Cover Designer: Harry Voigt
Copy Editor: Kristi McRae
Illustrator: Jennifer Johnson
Printer: Transcontinental Printing

Printed in Canada
1 2 3 4 5 6 7   04 03 02 01 00

Library of Congress Cataloging-in-Publication Data

Norton, Cheryl.
   Beginning Racquetball / Cheryl Norton, James E. Bryant.—5th ed.
     p. cm.
   Includes index.
   ISBN 0-534-57144-1
   1. Racquetball—Handbooks, manuals, etc. I. Bryant, James E. II.
    Title.

   GV1003.34 .N67 2001
   796.343—dc21

00-43973

Wadsworth/Thomson Learning
10 Davis Drive
Belmont, CA 94002-3098
USA

For more information about our products, contact us:
Thomson Learning Academic Resource Center
1-800-423-0563
http://www.wadsworth.com

International Headquarters
Thomson Learning
International Division
290 Harbor Drive, 2nd Floor
Stamford, CT 06902-7477
USA

UK/Europe/Middle East/South Africa
Thomson Learning
Berkshire House
168-173 High Holborn
London WC1V 7AA
United Kingdom

Asia
Thomson Learning
60 Albert Street, #15-01
Albert Complex
Singapore 189969

Canada
Nelson Thomson Learning
1120 Birchmount Road
Toronto, Ontario M1K 5G4
Canada

Contents

Preface

Beginning Racquetball is designed for the beginning player, the novice who is attempting to develop skills and knowledge in racquetball. More advanced players also can use this book to review skills and strategy. Actually, the book is a confirmation for more advanced players that their skills are consistent with fundamental play, and that they are making progress beyond the beginning level.

The changes in this fifth edition are subtle. The revised 2000 rules are included. Several new photographs and diagrams better characterize a specific skill or concept. We also have added new "cues," adjusted "Points to Remember," updated the section on equipment, expanded information on doubles play, and included a reference key when discussing rules.

Chapters 1 and 2 provide information on equipment, safety and resources, and preparation for playing the game. Chapters 3–5 introduce the preliminaries to the stroke in racquetball and various offensive and defensive strokes used in playing the game. These are the basic strokes that enable a player to engage in a competitive experience. Chapter 6 provides information on putting the ball in play. Chapter 7 introduces use of the back wall and corners of the racquetball court once the ball is in play. Chapters 8 and 9 provide insight on how to put all the strokes together in a plan for offensive and defensive strategy. Chapter 10 provides drills for practice. Chapter 11 is a summary of the basic rules and etiquette associated with racquetball.

The text will serve as a guide to develop the physical and mental skills necessary to succeed in racquetball. Photographs and illustrations present the concept of the game visually to aid in comprehending the skills of the game. The summary sections "Points to Remember" and "Common Errors and How to Correct Them" highlight key information, and the "Cues" inserts provide a conceptual view of the game. And, as a tool for assisting student self-evaluation, a set of Self Testing Questions exist at the end of each chapter. Overall the text establishes a solid primer of information and insight for racquetball players.

Acknowledgments

The contributions to the fifth edition of *Beginning Racquetball* are accumulative. Previous editions of the text have been supported by creative ideas, suggestions, and efforts from reviewers, models, and the illustrator. Over the course of five editions there are numerous people to specifically thank. They include photographers Greg Hazard and Eric Risberg, models Elida Shilts, Scott Foster, Lisa McLaws, and Brad Carter. A thank you is also extended to the San Jose Athletic Club (San Jose, California) and Schoeber's Athletic Club (Pleasanton, California) for site photographs, along with a special thank you to Cheryl Namoca, Schoeber's Activity Director for her able assistance in providing facilities, equipment and models.

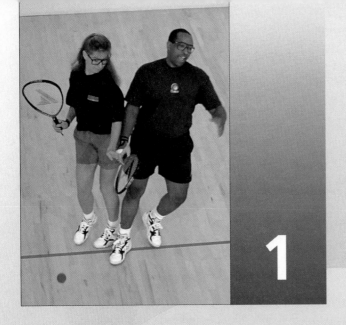

Court, Equipment, Safety, and Resources

Racquetball is played in an enclosed court using the four walls, floor, and ceiling as the playing surface. In areas where a four-wall court cannot be built, one- or three-wall racquetball may be played. The rules and strategy for all these games are similar. This text, however, will concentrate only on the more complex, four-wall game.

The dimensions and markings on the court are as shown in Figure 1.1.

Fortunately, the terminology used to describe the court is easily learned: floor, ceiling, front, back, and side walls. The floor lines identify the **service zone** (bounded by the service line and short line), two rectangular areas called **service boxes** and the drive serve lines. The only other mark on the court denotes the **receiving line** for the player returning the serve. The floor surface is also divided into playing areas to define

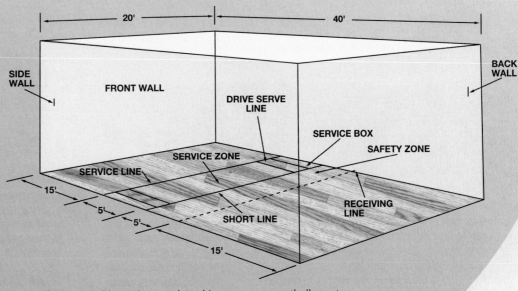

Figure 1.1 Dimensions and markings on a racquetball court.

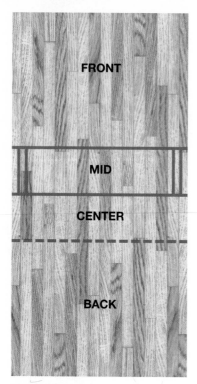

Figure 1.2 Designated floor areas on the court.

court positioning, as shown in Figure 1.2.

Racquetball was invented by Joe Sobek in 1949. Using a handball court, he combined the games of handball and squash into a paddle ball game, first called *paddle rackets,* that eventually evolved into today's game of racquetball. The game increased in popularity in the 1970s, and by the late 1970s and early 1980s it had become one of the fastest growing sports in America. At a point in the mid-1980s, racquetball declined in popularity, but by the late 1980s the decline had leveled off, and today the game has nearly 7.7 million American players. There is an overall ratio of 2:1 of male vs. female participants, and nearly 60% of all players are within the age group of 18–34. Racquetball is played in 89 countries. World Championships, the Pan American Games, and future Olympics are all part of the present and future of racquetball (American Sport Analysis, Inc., 1996).

Brief Overview of the Game

Racquetball is played as a best-of-three match. The object of the game is to score 15 points before your opponent does, and if each of you wins one game, to play a third game to 11 points. Only the serving player scores points. A point is scored when the server's opponent fails to hit the ball to the front wall before the ball touches the floor twice. If the server fails to return the ball to the

front wall, the server loses serve. In this way, service (and the opportunity to score) is alternated until one player or team accumulates 15 points (11 points in the third game), and wins the game.

Racquetball may be played with two (singles), three (cut-throat), or four (doubles) players. In singles, one player opposes another player, and in doubles, one two-person team plays another two-person team. In cut-throat, a single server plays against two opponents. When the server loses serve, one of the opponents becomes the server and plays against the remaining two players. Scoring is the same as in singles.

In all games, each rally (exchange of hits between opposing players) is begun with a **legal serve.** For the serve to be legal, the server must stand in the service zone, drop the ball to the floor, and strike it on the rebound so it hits the front wall before any other court surface. The receiver stands between the back of the safety zone line and the back wall in order to return the serve. To return the serve legally, the receiver must wait until the served ball passes the short line and either bounces in or crosses the safety zone. The front wall rebound may not touch the floor in front of or on the short line. Before the ball hits the floor, it may rebound off one side wall but not off the ceiling, back wall, or both side walls. The return of serve and any other hit, however, may rebound the ball off any surface except the floor before reaching the front wall. Service is changed when the server fails to keep the ball in play or he/she does not serve legally. If the receiver fails to return the ball to the front wall, a point is scored.

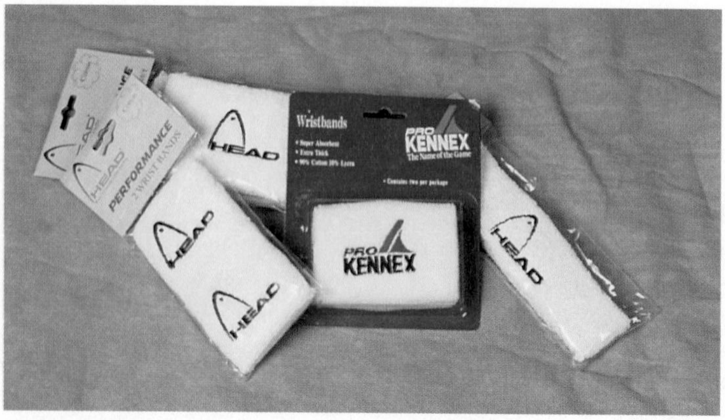

Outfitting for Play

Clothing

The usual dress for both men and women is a sports shirt or T-shirt and shorts.

Headbands and wristbands (see Figure 1.3) aid in absorbing of perspiration around the head and hands and are optional. Shirts will help to absorb body

Figure 1.3 Racquetball headbands and wristbands.

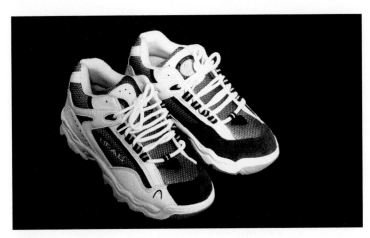

Figure 1.4 Racquetball court shoes.

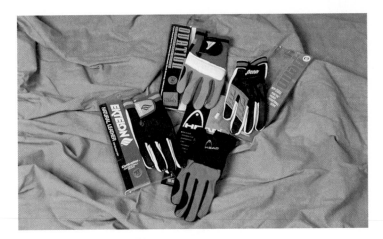

Figure 1.5 Racquetball gloves.

A court shoe should have excellent traction. Gum rubber soles provide that traction. Shoes should also have a full-length midsole for proper cushioning, ventilation, and lateral support. A reminder for proper footwear includes wearing athletic socks with your court shoe to prevent the foot from sliding in the shoe and creating blisters.

Gloves

The use of a glove is optional and dependent upon your comfort and need. Many players wear a glove on their racquet hand to help maintain a better grip on the racquet and prevent the racquet from slipping from their hand. Quality gloves will dry soft after use and will provide a firm grip to the racquet. High performance gloves are made of ultra thin graphite, Kevlar, and neoprene materials. These materials provide glove strength and durability, and padded protection for the knuckles from wall and floor impact. You should look for gloves that provide ventilation and good "feel" to the grip (see Figure 1.5).

Protective Eyewear

Players must wear protective eyewear designed specifically for racquetball players. Competitive rules require pre-tested eye guards that meet specific safety standards the United States Racquetball Association (USRA) provides through a list of approved eyewear from companies including Ektelon, ITECH, Leershot, Black Knight, Eagle Eyewear, and Leader. These competitive rules extend to the reputable management of any court facility. Lensed eyewear is now developed for the player who wears corrective lenses and the player who does not wear glasses. Severe eye damage, including detached retinas and the loss of vision, have followed direct eye hits with either the ball or the racquet. Proper protective eyewear dramatically reduces the possibility of eye injury (see Figure 1.6).

Basic features of protective eyewear require selecting a lens that is distortion-free and provides peripheral vision. Lenses are made of polycarbonate material and must be treated with anti-fog and hard coat treatment that

perspiration and must be worn at all times during play. Body perspiration dripping onto the floor of the court presents a potential hazard to cutting and turning associated with footwork.

Shoes

The footwear worn on a racquetball court should be an athletic shoe that supports shifting body weight and lateral movement on the court. Racquetball court shoes (see Figure 1.4) are made specifically for players who take the game seriously. A player also can wear tennis shoes or basketball shoes, but they are secondary alternatives to the court shoe. Shoes designed for running should never be used, and dark-soled shoes are also restricted, since they mar court surfaces. Technology has produced an ultra-lightweight court shoe that is designed as a ¾-top or low-cut shoe.

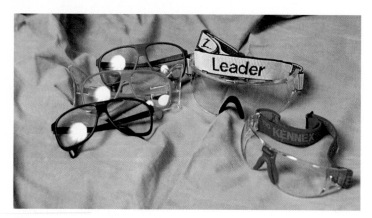

Figure 1.6 Protective eyewear.

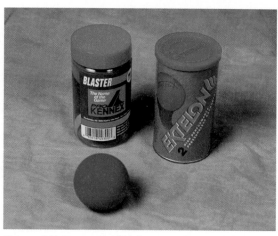

Figure 1.7 Racquetball balls.

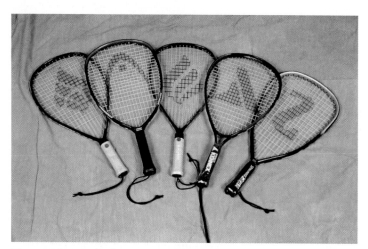

Figure 1.8 Longbody racquets — 22" length.

resists scratching, and the frame must be shock resistant.

Ball

Specifications for a racquetball ball are determined by the United States Racquetball Association. Balls come in several colors, but most are blue or, for competition, green (see Figure 1.7). They are 2¼ inches in diameter and weigh 1.6 ounces. When dropped from a 100-inch height at a temperature of 70–74 degrees, they should rebound 68 to 72 inches, or be replaced with a new ball.

Racquets

The selection of a racquet is dependent upon the style of play, skill level, and amount of money you want to invest. The frame of the racquet has previously been constructed of various materials

including aluminum, graphite, fiberglass, and boran. Most racquets today are made of graphite, high modulus graphite, ultra-high modulus graphite, Hype Carbon, Tri-Carbon, and titanium (see Figure 1.8). These advanced technologies contribute to racquets that have both power and control, plus reduced vibration. These graphite and graphite-composite racquets generate tremendous power.

Modern technology has not only developed advanced racquet frames of various composite materials that enhance play, but racquet sizes and shapes have also changed dramatically. Racquets are now produced from midsize to macro oversize. These sizes extend up to 107 square inches of racquet face, and are presently designed in teardrop or quadriform shapes. Racquets are designed to weigh as little as 5½ to 7 ounces, because the larger the hitting surface, the more need for the weight of the racquet to be light to maintain the ability to maneuver the racquet. All racquets have a very large "sweet spot" that is usually elongated and covers a larger width than the original conventional racquets. Racquet length now can be measured up to 22 inches, and these extra-length racquets are called longbodies.

Racquets are now designed with an extended racquet throat, and the larger racquet faces have longer *mainstrings*, which translates to more power. These larger racquet faces have longer strings, and the longer the string, the more it

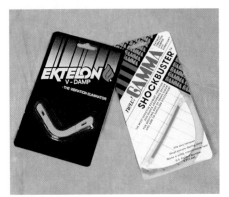

Figure 1.9 Accessories for racquets.

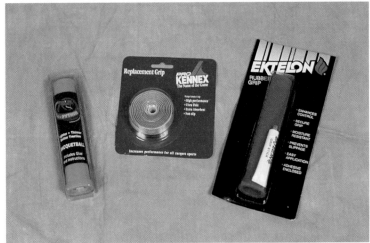

Figure 1.10 Accessories for racquet grip.

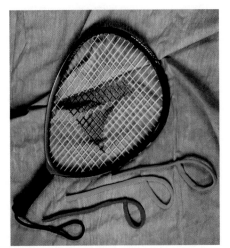

Figure 1.11 Replacement safety tether.

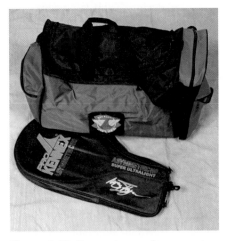

Figure 1.12 Bag and cover for racquet.

can stretch; consequently, the greater the trampoline effect, the greater the power. Racquets are strung with various gauges of string: thin gauge of 17 or 18 provides more power, a heavier gauge of 15 provides a little less power but more durability.

There are accessories for racquets (see Figure 1.9). As an example, tape can be affixed to the racquet to protect the bumper guards and strings from damage caused by striking the walls. In addition, dampening vibrators are woven through the strings of a racquet to reduce racquet vibration.

Grips and Grip Size

As a rule of thumb, the grip size should be smaller than that of a tennis racquet. Grip sizes range from super small to medium. Most experts suggest that when gripping the racquet properly, the middle finger of the racquet hand should just touch the palm at the base of the thumb, to allow for a good wrist snap and racquet control.

Racquet Strings and Tension

Racquets are often already strung when you buy them. When a racquet is strung or restrung, you need to specify the amount of tension. Tension levels are recommended in information accompanying a new racquet, but if you select a tension level, it should range from 25 to 50 pounds. On the average, players

opt for a tension level of 25–30 pounds. The less the string tension, the more control a player has, and the tighter the racquet is strung, the more power. The material used to string is usually monofilament nylon.

Handle and Tether

Racquet handle grips are made of rubber or leather. Although leather is more expensive if tack-treated, it usually allows you to grip the racquet more securely. When selecting a racquet, look for a handle that dampens vibration and reduces wrist fatigue. The racquet grip has an accessory designed for players who use gloves and players who don't use gloves. These "grippers" (see Figure 1.10) provide for a firm grip that enhances the stroke and also serves as a safety feature.

To be legal, each racquet must have a **tether** attached to the handle. The tether is a safety cord worn on the wrist during play. Replacement tethers (see Figure 1.11) may be purchased where racquetball equipment is supplied.

Racquets are easy to care for if you use some common sense. Try not to leave your racquet in the back seat of your car. Extremes in heat or cold will cause the strings to become brittle or break down faster. Keep a cover on the racquet to prevent objects from catching in the strings (see Figure 1.12). If the strings are breaking frequently, insert plastic eyelets where the string wraps around the frame to protect the strings from wearing on the edge and possibly prevent breaking. Or, make sure you string your racquet with a more durable 15-gauge string.

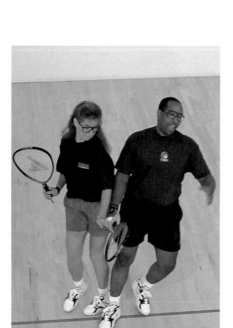

Figure 1.13 Hitting a ball when your opponent is in the way.

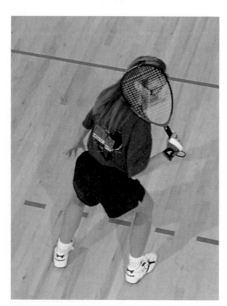

Figure 1.14 Protecting your face by looking through the racquet strings.

Safety

Safety During Play

Safety on the court begins when you walk onto the court, put on your protective eyewear, and shut the door to protect against people walking in during play. During play, a racquetball court is safe only if all the players are courteous. This means staying out of your opponent's path to the ball or arm swing. Similarly, no shot is "too good to pass up" if a player is in the path of your swing. There is no excuse for hitting another player with your racquet. If a player is so close to you that there is a risk of contact, then stop play rather than continuing (see Figure 1.13).

In addition, learn to play the strokes correctly. Too many players keep their tennis stroke alive in the racquetball court. Wide swings from the shoulder require the room a tennis court provides. There is no place on the racquetball court for this kind of play.

As mentioned, each racquet must have a tether or safety cord attached to it. This tether is worn around the wrist of the racquet hand to prevent the racquet from flying out of the player's hand and injuring someone on the court. This cord must be used at all times.

Positioning on the court when receiving serve is important. The receiver must remember to wait for the ball to bounce or pass beyond the short line of the safety zone before stepping into the zone to return the serve. By doing this, the server is protected from potential serious injury either by being hit by the receiver's racquet at contact with the ball or in the receiver's follow-through.

During play you should continually be aware of players' movements on the court. Stay out of the way of the player hitting the ball, and when it is your turn to hit, take your shot only if it is clear. Most balls are hit from the back of the court forward. If you are in front of the ball, DO NOT turn completely around to "see" what is going on behind you in the back court. This not only exposes your chest and abdomen to a hard-hit ball, but it also leaves your face unprotected. Rather, you should angle your body slightly so you can see the back court with your peripheral vision and hold the racquet to protect your face as you look through the strings.

Using the racquet to protect your face from an oncoming ball (see Figure 1.14) is an effective safety measure only if the racquet "beats" the ball to the target. Don't rely on your reflexes to get the racquet up in time to protect your face. As a precaution, you can use your racquet as a shield if your face is exposed to the ball's path, and you must always wear your protective eyewear to protect your eyes against the stray shot. This way, you can play the game and finish still looking the same as when you entered the court.

Experienced players will let the ball rebound off the back wall before playing it. This means that a center court position has to be held open for that player to follow the ball. Anticipate the most direct path to the ball that your opponent can take, and keep that court position clear. Racquetball is not a game that allows mental lapses. Each player must know where the ball is at all times, and where the other players are moving.

Should you interfere with your opponent's movement on the court, interfere with completion of that player's swing, or get hit by your opponent's racquet, a **hinder** must be called. A hinder should be called by the offended player in a recreational game and by a referee during tournament play. When a **dead-ball** hinder is called, play is stopped and the point is replayed from the serve. When an **avoidable hinder** is called, play is also stopped, but in this case a loss of rally by the offending player occurs. Contact does not have to occur for a hinder to be requested. Preferably, play should stop before players or racquets collide, to avoid potential injury (see Figure 1.15).

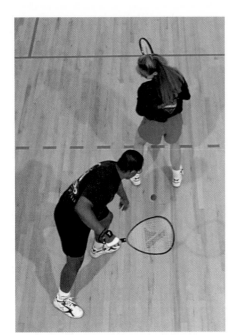

Figure 1.15 Player not leaving center court to give opponent clear shot off a back wall rebound.

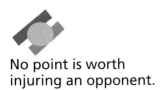

No point is worth injuring an opponent.

Safety is a matter of habit and thinking. Protect yourself by wearing protective eyewear, using your racquet as a shield, keeping your tether on your wrist, and closing the door of the court when playing. Anticipate your opponent's position, the path of the ball, and the movement of players on the court. Most important, remember that racquetball is just a game, and one point is not worth risking your well-being or that of your opponent just to make a shot.

Racquetball Injuries

Specific injuries are related to racquetball. A beginning player's injuries tend to be bruises caused by being struck by the ball or by an opponent's racquet, eye injuries from being struck by the ball, sprained ankles, pulled muscles, tendonitis, and blisters on the hands and feet. Most of the injuries result from playing in a small, confined space with another person who has a racquet in his or her hand. The predictability or unpredictability of an opponent's movement, along with the inexperience of a player, further creates the potential for injury. In addition, the game is designed for strenuous effort, and many individuals attempt to play without proper warm-up or adequate conditioning, compounding the possibility of injury.

Bruises are part of the game, and as long as a hematoma (severe bruising) does not develop, they are considered minor injuries. Wearing protective clothing, such as sweat pants and top, provides some protection from the potential of bruises caused by being struck by the ball. Court awareness assists in avoiding being hit by an opponent's racquet. Once a bruise, if minor, has formed, treatment usually consists of cold compresses or ice packs designed to reduce swelling and encourage faster healing.

Eye injuries can be serious. Following preventive safety measures, discussed earlier, is critical to avoiding this type of injury. The potential for internal damage to the eye, or a detached retina, is significant enough to encourage the preventive measure of wearing protective eyewear. If an eye injury is sustained, medical treatment must be given immediately.

Sprained ankles usually are caused by a player making a quick turn without the foot following in the turn, or by lack of awareness of the opponent's positioning, creating an unexpected foot movement. Muscle strains or pulls result from the same overextension, and improper warm-up and stretching. As with bruises, ice or cold compresses can reduce swelling of a sprained ankle or a strain or muscle pull, speeding up recovery. A major caution regarding these types of injuries: Make sure you have suffered only a minor sprain rather than ligament or tendon damage or a broken bone, as more severe injuries obviously require a totally different application of treatment.

Tendonitis affecting the elbow usually is caused by too much vibration in the racquet at contact with the ball, too many hours of play without rest, or incorrect mechanics when executing a backhand stroke. Tendonitis also is found in the shoulder area. This usually is caused by incorrect stroke mechanics or extensive playing time without rest. These injuries, characterized by inflammation of the elbow or shoulder joint, require rest to heal. In some instances an elbow support or splint can be used as a preventive measure for elbow tendonitis, but nothing replaces proper stroke mechanics in avoiding this type of injury.

Achilles tendon injuries also occur in racquetball. Jumping and landing on the ball of the foot without lowering the heel, or pushing off the ball of the foot, placing extreme pressure on the tendon, can cause it to rupture. The tendon rupturing sounds like a gunshot report, and the player becomes immediately immobile. Ridged, high-arched feet with heels that angle inward, or flat feet that roll inward, are more vulnerable to Achilles tendon problems. Players often ignore chronic soreness of the Achilles and continue to play. The Achilles tendon and the sheath that surrounds it become inflamed, and soreness, swelling, and pain result. Ignoring these signs can cause severe problems. The only way to address the injury is to stop playing and rest.

Prevention includes stretching as part of warm-up and warm-down. Orthotics for your shoe is another preventive measure, but elevating your heel also shortens the tendon, when what is needed is to lengthen the tendon. As a result, stretching becomes even more important as a preventive measure. A stiff or achy Achilles tendon is a sign of impending rupture. Rest and consultation with a sports medicine professional are recommended to address the problem.

Blisters are common in most sport participation situations. They usually can be avoided in racquetball. Blisters are caused by moisture, pressure, or friction. Hand blisters are caused by an improper grip size and extensive play that causes a "hot spot" on the hand. This type of blister can be avoided by proper racquet grip sizing and by wearing a racquetball glove during play.

Blisters that develop on the feet, due to friction, usually are caused by the feet sliding in the shoe. To address this situation, wear a pair of cotton socks with insoles as a preventive measure. Using appropriate shoes designed for court play also go a long way in preventing blisters. Once blisters have developed, the main concern is to make sure they do not get infected. For a foot blister, an athletic trainer can create a doughnut-shaped pad to reduce the pain at the pressure point, and allow you to continue to play.

Racquetball requires quick turns, stops and starts. Repetitive twisting and trunk rotation are a part of racquetball. The risk of back injury is increased because of the movement required in the game. Preventive measures include a total conditioning program, proper stretching (see Chapter 2), and sound stroke technique.

From an injury standpoint, there is also the danger of dehydration, as well as cramps that can make participation in racquetball uncomfortable. Racquetball courts often do not have good air circulation; consequently the environment can become very warm. Intake of liquids will assist in avoiding cramps and dehydration. (Chapter 2 provides further information on fluid intake.)

If you follow safety procedures, your racquetball experience not only will be relatively injury-free, but also will be more enjoyable. If an injury does occur, immediate attention to the injury will hasten your recovery.

Resources

A multitude of resources is available in racquetball for your use. The United States Racquetball Association (USRA) is the national association that provides the official rules and publishes a bimonthly magazine entitled *RACQUETBALL Magazine* for its members. In addition, the USRA produces instructional materials, and provides insurance for racquetball competitors. The USRA sanctions age-group and various skill-level tournaments, sponsors regional associations, trains and certifies players and instructors, and generally promotes racquetball at the grassroots level. One of its noteworthy efforts is the promotion of racquetball for disabled athletes, including those who use a wheelchair and individuals who have visual and hearing impairments. The USRA offers a membership for tournament competitors, and for non-competitors provides the *RACQUETBALL Magazine* subscription option.*

Resources also include professional instruction and coaching. Nearly every college and university offers racquetball as a course for students. In addition, fitness and sports clubs usually have a professional instructor available for lessons, along with a series of racquetball functions that include local tournaments

---

* The USRA requires a $20 fee for a competitive membership and a $15 charge for the magazine. The membership application address is: USRA, 1685 West Uintah, Colorado Springs, CO 80904-2906 or www.usra.org.

for all ages and skill levels. When taking racquetball lessons, questions you should ask of an instructor include:

■ How much individual time will you provide me? (The more individual time, the better.)

■ What will you teach me? (You need to develop as a player rather than repeat past learning experiences.)

■ What kind of teaching credentials do you have? (Anyone can attempt to teach racquetball, but USRA instructor status or a teaching credential associated with racquetball is critical.)

Countless equipment manufacturers support racquetball, contributing to your racquetball development. Ektelon is a good example of a corporation that not only produces excellent equipment, but provides instructional materials on how to play racquetball. Local companies also support development of the game. The Internet provides many additional resources. Courtesy Sports, a marketing company for racquetball, has a web site address of: www.courtesy sports.com. If you are interested in ordering instructional video tapes on racquetball, you can access: www. masterball.com and find three video tapes entitled *Mastery of Racquetball— Doubles, Mastery of Racquetball—The Complete Success Program* (*Singles*), and *Think Fast . . . Fitness, Agility and Speed Training.* There are countless other racquetball web sites, most providing information on equipment or instruction, that you can access by simply entering the key word *racquetball.*

Points to Remember

➜ **Do** put on your protective eyewear before entering the court.

➜ **Do** shut the door to the court before you begin hitting.

➜ **Do** be courteous to all players on the court.

➜ **Do** use proper strokes to hit the ball, and avoid swinging wildly.

➜ **Do** keep the tether of the racquet securely on your wrist.

➜ **Do** know where the ball is at all times.

➜ **Do** remember that racquetball is just a GAME!

➜ **Do** remember that winning a point is never worth injuring an opponent.

➜ **Don't** swing at the ball if your opponent is in the way.

➜ **Don't** get in the way of another player who is hitting the ball.

➜ **Don't** turn completely around to see what is going on behind you.

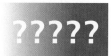

Self Testing Questions

Answers to Self Testing Questions are located on page 131.

1. A legal match score is:
   a. 15–13, 7–15, 15–10
   b. 21–17, 21–3
   c. 13–15, 15–6, 11–10
   d. 13–15, 15–13, 15–14

2. A legal serve includes the following:
   a. Server stands in the service zone. After the server bounces the ball and strikes it, the ball must hit the front wall first, and then clear the short line and bounce before striking a second wall.
   b. Server stands in the service zone. After the server bounces the ball and strikes it, the ball must hit the front wall first, and then clear the short line, striking no more than one side wall before bouncing on the floor.
   c. Server stands in the service zone. After the server bounces the ball and strikes it, the ball must hit the front wall first, and then clear the short line before striking the back wall.
   d. Server stands in the service zone. After the server bounces the ball and strikes it, the ball may hit one side wall before hitting the front wall, and then clear the short line before striking the floor.

3. The receiver of serve may return the serve by
   a. contacting the ball and striking a side wall and front wall followed by the ball making contact with the floor.
   b. contacting the ball and striking the ceiling and front wall followed by the ball making contact with the floor.
   c. contacting the ball and striking the front wall followed by the ball making contact with the floor.
   d. all of the above.

4. When the ball has been placed into play it may be
   a. hit on the fly.
   b. hit after it bounces once.
   c. hit after two bounces.
   d. both a and b.

5. Shirts must be worn because they
   a. look good.
   b. absorb sweat.
   c. provide the opponent with visual contact.
   d. all of the above.

6. Characteristics of quality protective eyewear include
   a. polycarbonate material.
   b. non-scratch lenses.
   c. non-fog lenses.
   d. all of the above.

7. The modern racquetball racquets are made of
   a. aluminum.
   b. fiberglass.
   c. graphite or composite.
   d. wood.

8. List four significant rules that are reflective of safe play:

   _____

   _____

   _____

   _____

   _____

   _____

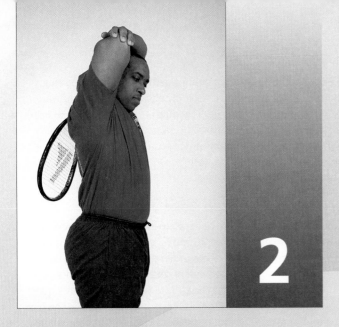

2

Preparation for Play

**Use it
or lose it.**

Racquetball players cannot use their skills and strategy to the best advantage if they do not maintain proper physical conditioning. With less-than-optimal fitness, fatigue sets in too quickly, injuries are more likely to occur, and the quality of play declines. Although the optimal level of fitness for each player is an individual decision based upon the quality of play he or she wants to maintain, conditioning for all levels of play must be a year-round activity.

Physical conditioning is not like riding a bicycle (once you have it, you never lose it). Instead, the state of conditioning is transient and responds only to the amount of use or disuse of the body. If the body is not "used" with exercise, it loses the capabilities, such as strength and endurance, that exercise promotes. This is not to imply that physical conditioning will help improve your racquetball skills. If you want to be a better racquetball player, you must play racquetball. Optimal conditioning, however, will allow you to get the *best* out of your skills.

Some aspects of physical conditioning should be trained on a weekly basis regardless of whether or not you are playing racquetball. Thus, when play begins, you are ready to play your best. Most people make the mistake of trying to condition for a sport at the same time they are starting to play. This increase in activity overloads the body and the body "breaks down." Either an actual injury occurs or general fatigue takes away the pleasure of the game. Ideally, the racquetball player should always be "fit" to play. Minimally, to be fit means that you have conditioned your body aerobically and with weight training.

Aerobic Conditioning for Recovery

Although success in racquetball relies on quickness, skill, and strategy, none of these factors will be important if you are too tired to move. During rallies, most of the energy the body uses is a product of anaerobic metabolism, the release of energy without the use of oxygen.

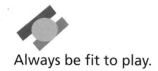

Always be fit to play.

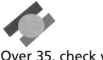

Over 35, check with your physician.

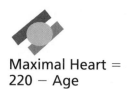

Maximal Heart =
220 − Age

Restoring these energy supplies for the next rally, however, requires use of oxygen. Therefore, although energy needs during play are not primarily aerobic ("with oxygen"), the more oxygen that can be inhaled between rallies, the faster you can recover and the less tired you will become during the game. This means that part of your physical conditioning program must involve aerobic conditioning—training to bring oxygen into the body, circulate it to the muscles, and utilize it efficiently to recover quickly.

Before beginning any aerobic conditioning program, you should make sure it is safe for your body. As a general rule, if you are under 35, have had a thorough physical in the last year, and have no reason to suspect you are not healthy, you can begin exercising immediately. If you have not had a medical checkup in over a year, suspect that you may be suffering from hypertension or diabetes, are extremely overweight (more than 20 percent over your suggested weight), use tobacco products, or have other health problems (such as back problems), check with your physician before starting an aerobic conditioning program.

If you are over 35, you should have medical clearance from your physician. Make sure your physician understands the type of program in which you want to get involved. If you obtain clearance, you are ready to begin.

You can use a variety of activities to train your body aerobically: walking, running, cross-country skiing, swimming, and bicycling, as well as aerobic exercise classes (dance, bench stepping, and so on). These activities are good conditioners because performing them successfully requires large amounts of oxygen to be brought into the body, which allows your system to literally "practice" oxygen utilization. Although any of these activities may be used, a jog-run program is suggested because racquetball requires you to run around the court. Just going out for a brisk walk may or may not be helpful in improving your conditioning for this sport. For aerobic conditioning to occur, certain guidelines must be followed. These guidelines define how hard you must exercise (intensity), how long (duration), and how often (frequency) for the exercise to be safe, yet hard enough for training to result.

Intensity

In general, the intensity of exercise is monitored by your heart rate. For most people under age 35, exercising between 70 percent and 85 percent of their maximal heart rate will provide an adequate intensity. Maximal heart rate is the maximal speed your heart can beat when exercising as hard as you can. One way to predict your maximal heart rate is to take 220 and subtract your age. After you have determined this number, simply calculate 70 percent and 85 percent of this number. This formula gives your exercise heart rate range. For example, a man who is 28 years old would have a predicted maximal heart rate of 192 (220 minus 28). His exercise heart rate range would be 134 (70 percent) to 163 (85 percent) beats per minute. Ideally, to train aerobically, your heart must be beating at a speed within this range.

For individuals between 35 and 50 years of age, the range is slightly different. Exercising between 60 percent and 70 percent of your maximal heart rate is a good place to begin. Because activity levels in this group are so variable, you can work at a higher intensity after several exercise sessions if you are in good aerobic condition and if the lower intensity seems too easy. To make sure you are not exercising above your capabilities, use the "talking test" as a guide. During aerobic conditioning, you should be able to talk and exercise at the same time. If you cannot, your effort is too hard and you are not bringing in enough oxygen to match the exercise intensity. This means *slow down*. If you find 60 percent to 70 percent too hard, slow to a lower level. As conditioning progresses, you will be able to move into the higher exercise heart rate range. Give yourself time to condition for it.

Finally, individuals over age 50 should begin at an intensity between 50 percent and 60 percent of their

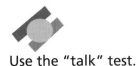

Use the "talk" test.

predicted maximal heart rate. Again, use the talk test as your guide, and regulate your exercise accordingly.

To check your heart rate, exercise for at least 5 minutes, then stop and take a 10-second count of your heartbeat. Use the pulse in your neck at the carotid artery, or the pulse at your wrist. Count the first beat you feel in the 10-second count as 0. At the end of the time period, multiply the number of beats counted by 6 to see if the equivalent beats per minute falls within the exercise heart rate range. If it is above the range, slow down. If it is below, speed up, unless the talk test suggests otherwise.

Duration

Now that you are working at the proper intensity, how long must you exercise at this level? Anywhere between 15 and 60 minutes will provide enough time to give your body sufficient practice at using oxygen. In general, 20 to 30 minutes is recommended as the proper exercise duration. This means 20 to 30 minutes of constant, nonstop exercise at your exercise heart rate. If this level of activity is too difficult for you to begin with, start with a jog-walk interval program. Begin by jogging a few minutes, and then walk until you are ready to jog again. Keep track of the time you spent jogging versus walking. Each week, try to increase the amount of time jogging and decrease the walking time until you can jog the entire 20 minutes. Don't be afraid to jog slowly. This is a conditioning activity, not a race!

Frequency

How often should you do aerobic conditioning? Three to four times a week is ideal and five times is tolerated well. Participating in more than five aerobic exercise sessions a week may result in an increased rate of injuries to muscles and joints.

For the exercise sessions to be of most value, give yourself between 24 and 48 hours rest between each aerobic

workout. The more out of shape you are, the more recovery time you will need. If your recovery time is longer than 48 hours, some detraining in aerobic conditioning will occur. Therefore, keep your program regular in frequency but sensible in stress in order to balance your exercise needs with your capabilities.

Aerobic conditioning should be a base for all your sports programs and, as such, should be done consistently throughout the year. When you are playing more racquetball, however, you may find that you have to cut back on aerobic conditioning because of time constraints or energy limitations. Cutting back to two exercise sessions a week will just maintain aerobic conditioning without developing it. Therefore, if you must decrease your aerobic exercise, maintain at least two aerobic sessions a week to completely avoid detraining in this capacity. Your heart won't get any stronger, but at least you should minimize deconditioning. Developing your physical condition takes time and effort, but you have the rest of your life to work at it.

Weight Training: Developing Strength and Endurance

Muscular strength and endurance help provide power to your racquetball stroke. Without adequate "muscle" behind each shot, the speed of the ball will be compromised. Muscular endurance helps to maintain this power during long rallies or through a prolonged match. These two muscle capabilities go hand in hand and should be developed simultaneously to get the most benefit for play.

One of the best ways to develop strength and endurance is through weight training. For racquetball, this training should be concentrated on the muscles of the arms, shoulders, chest,

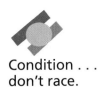

Condition . . . don't race.

All recovery is aerobic.

Weight train for power in your stroke.

Learn proper lifting techniques.

upper back, abdominals, and legs. How do you know if you have adequate strength in these muscles?

1. Do you fail to hit the ball consistently as hard as you want, given that your technique is proper?
2. Do your legs get tired, especially after a long rally?

If your answer to either question is "yes," weight training may be helpful in improving the quality of your game. Before beginning a weight training program, follow the same precautions given for aerobic conditioning, and check with your physician to determine if this is a safe activity for you.

To improve strength and endurance, weight training should be done two to three times a week (preferably on the days you are not training aerobically). Ideally, when you are not playing racquetball weekly, you should concentrate on improving your strength through two or three workouts per week. During your racquetball season, you can maintain strength with one hard workout a week. Unlike aerobic conditioning, strength gains are retained for a longer time and don't require that you exercise as often to prevent detraining.

The question, then, is which weight training exercises will be most helpful for playing racquetball? The following is a general list of exercises that are beneficial for strengthening the muscles needed to play:

> Chest Press
> Abdominal Crunch
> Leg Press
> Upright Rowing
> Bent-Arm Pullover
> Leg Curl
> Shoulder Press
> Wrist Curls
> Leg Extension
> Triceps Extension

Each exercise should be done with 8 to 10 repetitions for 3 sets. Begin by using a weight that fatigues you to exhaustion in the third set. When you can complete this number of lifts comfortably, you can either increase the weight lifted (to increase strength) or increase the

number of repetitions per set (to increase endurance).

To learn lifting techniques and safety concerns, purchase a beginning weight training book at your local college bookstore. Books used by a college weight training class typically have excellent hints about weight training effectively and safely. If you still have questions, go to a supervised weight training room and ask for help.

If you do not have access to a weight training room, calisthenics can be valuable in increasing muscular strength and endurance. Exercises such as push-ups, crunches, and chin-ups, done in sets similar to weight training, will provide a good stimulus for strengthening. You can begin with 5 sets of 10 repetitions each. Rest 30 to 60 seconds between sets. If this level of exercise is too easy, increase the number of repetitions per set, rather than the number of sets, until you find a challenging routine.

Stair climbing or bench-stepping can be beneficial in developing leg strength. If you are running up a stairway, give yourself three times as long to recover as it took to run the stairs. For example, if you completed the stairs in 10 seconds, wait 30 seconds before repeating the climb. Repeat the stairs as many times as your condition allows.

When stepping on a bench, step up and down with one leg, repeating the movement 10 to 15 times, then switch legs. You may or may not need to rest when switching legs, depending on your condition. Try to complete 5 sets with each leg.

Improvement in strength and endurance takes time, but if you stay with it, your racquetball will improve simply because you are in better condition to play. Just being in good condition will not help if you do not prepare yourself physically and mentally to play before you enter the court. It is just as important to warm up your "engine" before a racquetball game as it is to keep yourself in good condition.

Points to Remember

→ Condition your body to play racquetball using aerobic activities and weight training exercises.

→ If you are over 35 or have a medical problem, check with your physician before you begin any strenuous exercise program.

→ To condition aerobically, monitor your intensity and exercise 20–30 minutes, three or four times a week.

→ Do weight training two or three times a week using muscles that racquetball skills require.

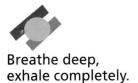

Breathe deep, exhale completely.

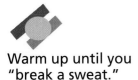

Warm up until you "break a sweat."

The Warm-Up

Whenever you are beginning to exercise, a rule of thumb is "never take your body by surprise." A **warm-up** to prepare yourself mentally and physically allows your body to shift gears smoothly from inactivity to activity. Without a warm-up, the stress of sudden activity can cause your body to rely on reserve energy sources normally used only during emergencies. Using your reserve energy at the start of the exercise can cause you to fatigue more quickly and adversely affect your level of play.

The warm-up should consist of three phases: *relaxation*, *increased heart activity*, and *stretching*. Relaxation is needed to relieve internal stress. The body responds to stress by increasing muscle tension. Tight muscles work in opposition to the free and fluid movement needed for any exercise or sport activity. In addition, any stretching exercises you may do will be more effective if the muscles are relaxed first. To relax, try sitting comfortably with your eyes closed for several minutes. Concentrate only on your breathing, remembering to exhale completely.

The second phase of the warm-up should increase your heart rate. This activity also will speed up the release of the body's available energy. As a result, at the beginning of the game, the reserve energy stores are not utilized. Playing racquetball will feel more comfortable, and you will not tire as rapidly.

Stair-stepping, cycling, running in place, and rope-skipping are examples of activities that will increase your heart rate. These activities should be done at low to moderate intensity. Your breathing should increase but never to the point of being out of breath. This phase of the warm-up is finished when you begin to "break a sweat," usually in 3–5 minutes.

Now that the body is warm, you can begin the last phase of the warm-up, stretching. Stretching is important to increase your ease and range of movement, referred to as **flexibility**. Although racquetball shots ideally should be hit just below waist level, there are opportunities for overhead strokes and returns when you must extend your arm to reach a ball. Flexibility in the shoulder joint will allow these movements to be done comfortably.

In addition, a player needs freedom of movement through the back to twist and turn, and through the hips and legs to bend and squat. If muscles are tight, movement is limited, detracting from your ability to reach the ball in different parts of the court with different strokes. Stretching exercises can ensure that you maintain the maximum range of movement in the joints of your body.

Ideally, stretching exercises should be done every day. If you are going to play racquetball, however, stretching should be included as part of your warm-up before play and cool-down afterward. Stretching before play helps to loosen the joints and muscles to

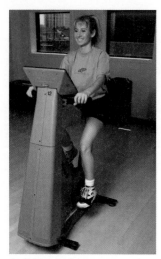
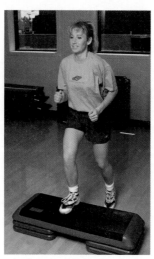
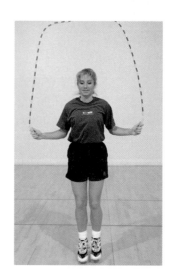
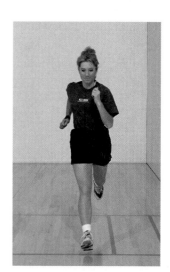

Activities to increase your heart rate before beginning to play.

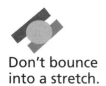

**Don't bounce
into a stretch.**

prepare for fast movements of the body during the game. After play, as you are cooling down, stretching helps to relieve contractions in fatigued muscles and prevent tight muscles the next day.

The stretching exercises presented here by no means comprise an exhaustive list of all exercises that can be done. Your favorites may be missing. Add them if they are helpful to you. The following stretches, however, do involve all major muscles used when playing racquetball. The basis for most of these stretches is extrapolated from Werner W. K. Hoeger's *Lifetime Physical Fitness & Wellness: A Personalized Program* (Morton Publishing, 1998).

Whichever exercises you do, several basic rules should be followed. Start with the head and work down the body, stretching the large muscles first and then the small muscles. Never

bounce into a stretched position. Trying to "force" a stretch contracts the muscle instead of allowing it to lengthen. Obviously, this is contrary to the purpose of the stretch. To avoid contracting the muscle, hold the stretch position without moving (except to breathe). This static position will allow the muscle to relax and lengthen. Once the muscle is relaxed during a stretch, you may want to try to stretch the muscle further to increase your range of motion.

Each static stretch should last at least 15 seconds and be repeated 3 to 5 times. This means that completing the set of stretching exercises will take a minimum of 10–15 minutes. If you choose to go back and repeat some exercises, plan on spending more time working on your flexibility rather than skipping other stretches. If you are excessively sore the next morning after

Stretching Exercises

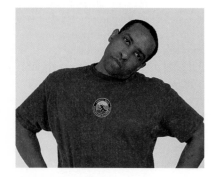
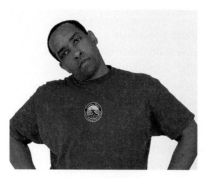

Lateral Head Tilt
Action: Tilt the head slowly and gently to one side. Pull down with the opposite shoulder. Hold the stretch 15 seconds. Alternate to the other side. Repeat as needed.
Areas stretched: Flexors and extensors, and ligaments of the cervical spine.

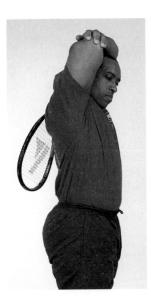

Shoulder and Arm Stretch

Action: Place the racquet head in the small of the back with the elbow in an up position. Place the non-racquet hand above the elbow and apply minimal pressure downward to place the shoulder area on stretch. Hold the stretch 15 seconds. Repeat as needed. (NOTE: you can do this same stretch with your non-racquet arm to relieve tension in this area.)

Areas stretched: Ligaments of the shoulder joint and triceps muscle.

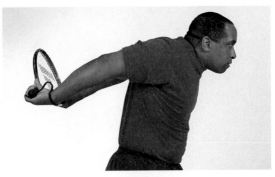

Shoulder Hyperextension Stretch

Action: Grasp the throat of the racquet with hands close together. Slowly bring the arms up to as close to a perpendicular position to the body as possible. Hold the stretch 15 seconds. Repeat as needed.

Areas stretched: Deltoid and pectoral muscles and ligaments of the shoulder joint.

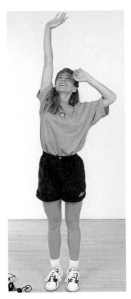

Ladder Climb

Action: While standing straight and looking up, alternately reach as high as possible with each arm. Hold the stretched position for 15 seconds before changing arms. Repeat as needed.

Areas stretched: Shoulder girdle and upper back muscles.

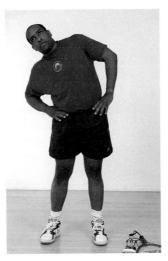

Side Stretch

Action: Stand with feet spread to shoulder width and hands on hips. Without moving the feet, or bending at the knees or hips, lean to one side. Do not bend forward. Hold stretch for 15 seconds. Repeat to the other side. Repeat as needed.

Areas stretched: Intercostal muscles and ligaments of the rib cage, muscles and ligaments of pelvis.

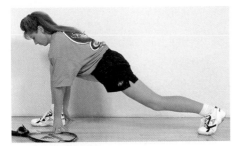

Groin Stretch

Action: Place one foot between hands, placed on floor, shoulder width apart. Lean forward with back leg stretched as far as possible. Try to keep forward leg bent at 90° angle. Hold 15 seconds. Switch legs. Repeat as needed.

Areas stretched: Groin and hip flexor muscles and ligaments.

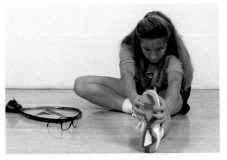

Modified Hurdler's Stretch

Action: On floor with one leg extended and sole of other foot touching inner thigh, slowly reach as far forward as possible. Pull upper body down. Hold 15 seconds. Repeat as needed.

Areas stretched: Hamstrings and lower back muscles, lumbar spine ligaments.

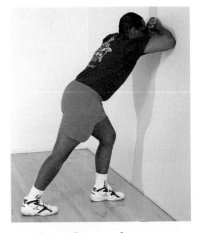

Heel Cord Stretch

Action: Stand 2–3 feet away from a wall. Stretch the heel of the back foot downward. Hold 15 seconds. Alternate feet. Repeat as needed.

Areas stretched: Achilles tendon, gastrocnemius and soleus muscles.

Stretch slowly . . . and hold for 15 seconds

Warm up until you "break a sweat."

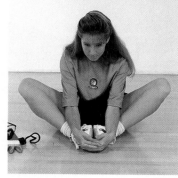

Butterfly

Action: Sit on floor with soles of your feet touching. Place your feet as close to your body as possible. Pull your trunk toward the floor. Hold 15 seconds. Repeat as needed.

Areas stretched: Lower back and spine, hip adductor muscles.

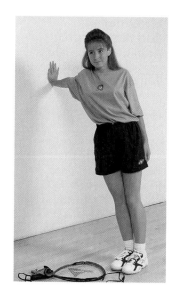

Forearm and Shoulder Stretch

Action: Stand arm's length away from wall. Place palm of hand on wall at shoulder height. Rotate shoulder forward while keeping hand in place. Hold 15 seconds. Alternate hands. Repeat as needed.

Areas stretched: Deltoid, biceps, forearm flexor muscles and forearm ligaments.

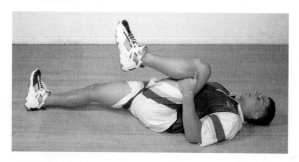

Single Knee to Chest Stretch

Action: Lie flat on padded surface. Bend one leg and place both hands on the hamstring side of the thigh. Pull this leg toward your chest. Try to keep head and back on the floor. Hold 15 seconds. Change legs. Repeat as needed.

Areas stretched: Lower back and hamstring muscles, and lumbar spine ligaments.

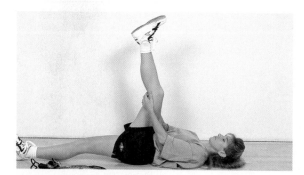

Hamstring Stretch

Action: Lying on floor with one leg extended and slightly bent, elevate opposite leg straight into the air. With both hands, gently pull on hamstring, bringing the leg closer to the upper body. Hold 15 seconds. Alternate legs, and repeat as needed.

Areas stretched: Lower back and lumbar spine ligaments, hamstring muscle.

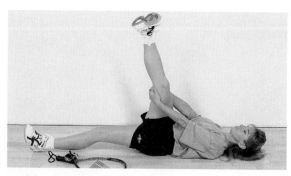

Ankle Stretch

Action: Using the same position needed for the Hamstring Stretch, alternately turn toes of elevated foot inward, then outward. Hold each position 15 seconds. When finished, slowly rotate your ankle through these positions. Alternate feet. Repeat as needed.

Areas stretched: Muscles and ligaments of the ankle and lower leg.

Focus, concentrate, and be mentally tough.

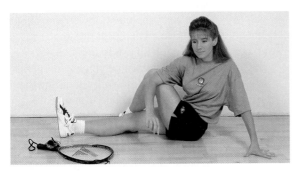

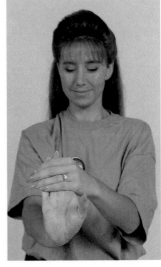

Trunk Twist

Action: Sit on floor and bend your left leg, placing your left foot on the outside of your right knee. Place your right elbow on your left knee and push against it. At the same time, try to rotate the trunk to the left (counterclockwise). Hold 15 seconds. Change to the other side. Repeat as needed.
Areas stretched: Lateral side of hip and trunk; trunk and lower back.

Wrist and Forearm Stretch

Action: Holding your left hand against your right hand, gently pull back against your fingers. Hold 15 seconds, then push your fingers down. Hold 15 seconds. Reverse hands and stretch. Repeat as needed.
Areas stretched: Forearm flexors and extensor muscles, wrist ligaments.

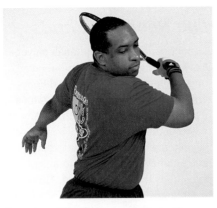

Serving Motion and Rotation

Action: With your racquet in your hand and arm extended in front of you, pull your arm through an arc and rotate your body until the racquet is directly behind you. Hold this position. Come forward slowly with the racquet as if stroking a ball, rotating your body forward. Complete the "swing" with a follow-through of the stroke. Turn your body as far as possible to exaggerate the follow-through, and hold this position 15 seconds. Repeat as needed.
Areas stretched: Hip, abdominal, chest, back, neck, and shoulder muscles; hip and spinal ligaments.

playing, stretch your sore muscles periodically throughout the day. Many of the following stretches can be done in street clothes, sitting in a chair, or even standing up.

If the more you stretch, the more sore the muscle becomes, STOP! You may be dealing with an injury rather than a tight muscle. Persistent or increasing pain is a signal that you should rest or even see a doctor.

The three warm-up phases should be done in sequence immediately before entering the court to play. Many people make the mistake of warming up and then waiting 5–10 minutes before playing racquetball. Consequently, most of the effect of the warm-up is lost. The increase in heart rate will decline within 1 to 2 minutes after the warm-up is over. Therefore, no time should be wasted getting onto the court.

Mental Readiness

Racquetball is played in an enclosed area with at least one other competitor. The game often can be played as a power game with the potential for intimidation. Unless your mind is focused on your game and skill execution rather than on your opponent, you will not perform at your best. More importantly, when in the court, this is a time to forget about your work, ignore outside noises and distractions, and eliminate self-doubt about your play. It is a time to be mentally ready to play. Mental readiness includes being focused on the court, concentrating on shots, and displaying mental toughness during the game.

Focus

The physical warm-up completed prior to play is intended to help your mind and body prepare for your time on the court. This preparation is wasted unless

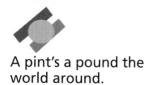

A pint's a pound the world around.

you can focus your thoughts on the game ahead rather than what happened yesterday or where you need to be after you finish play. Remember, you have chosen this game! Enjoy it by focusing all senses (i.e., hearing, touch, smell) on the environment you are in, a racquetball court! Not only will this allow you to enjoy the game more, but it will help you to play better because you won't be distracted. For the time you are in the court, that is your world!

Concentration

Concentration allows you to execute shots to the best of your ability. If you want to improve your game, you must think about what you are doing on the court. Well-executed shots just don't occur, they are a result of purposeful action. You must continue to concentrate on the action in the game as long as the rally continues. Don't congratulate yourself on a well-placed shot before the point is over. Think about where to place your next shot and mentally stay in the play until it is completed. Losing your concentration on the court not only prevents you from playing your best, but can also lead to injury if you lose the sense of where your opponent is positioned on the court. If you are having trouble maintaining concentration, try to relax by taking several deep breaths. Focus on the exhale of each breath and re-center your thoughts to this moment in time, not to what just happened. Give yourself a few encouraging words and constructive advice (i.e., I need to prepare earlier for my shot, keep moving my feet on the court). Concentrate on what will help you play better, not your frustrations at your mistakes.

Mental Toughness

As previously stated, racquetball, especially at the beginner's level, is often played as a power game. Hitting the ball hard, rather than ball placement, often becomes the immediate goal. As a result, it is not uncommon for beginning players to be hit with the ball during play. Also, beginning players don't always execute all shots correctly. Skill

improvement is part of learning! To play your best, you cannot allow the power of the opponent's shot, the pain of being hit by an errant ball, or your own frustration with your play get in the way of continuing to build your skill level. Hiding in the corner of the court because of fear of your opponent or worrying about whether you will repeat the same mishit will not help you to improve your game. Recognize that you are learning the game, visualize yourself hitting the ball perfectly, and eagerly anticipate your next opportunity to hit a winning shot! Above all, don't give up! Play every point hard, learn from your mistakes, and avoid losing control of your temper. If your opponent thinks that you have been "conquered" mentally, that will only provide a positive reinforcement for more aggressive play on his/her part.

The more you can stay calm during play, focus on the world in the court, and concentrate on your shots and the play of your opponent, the better opportunity you will have to play your best. After all, isn't this your primary goal?

The Need for Fluids

Another concern of racquetball players is overheating and dehydration. Prolonged **hyperthermia** (elevated body temperature) may lead to heat cramps, heat exhaustion, and heatstroke. Any of these conditions can arise when you are playing in a hot court for an extended time and have lost large amounts of body fluids through sweating. Although heat cramps are painful and temporarily disabling, they are not life-threatening. Untreated heatstroke, however, may be fatal.

To prevent problems associated with **dehydration** and overheating, make sure your clothing allows for good air circulation around your body. Avoid clothing that traps heat and promotes excessive sweating. This causes you to lose more body fluids than the exercise requires. Body fluids are important in regulating body temperature. If too many fluids are lost, your body is likely to overheat just like the radiator of your car when its water level is low. Some

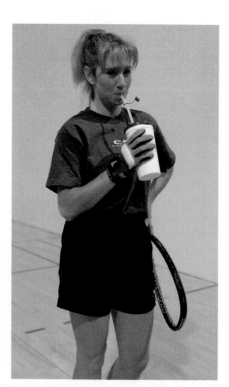

Start each game with a drink of water.

sweating is necessary to keep the body cool, however. Thus, the key to successful participation in a hot environment is to maintain an adequate level of body fluids by drinking.

To determine how much water to drink, a rule of thumb is "a pint's a pound the world around." For every pound of weight lost during exercise, you should drink a pint of water. To determine this amount, weigh yourself before and after playing, and drink a pint of water for each pound difference.

If you will be playing racquetball for more than 30 minutes, you should start replacing body fluids even before you begin the activity. Cold water (50° Fahrenheit) is best to drink when taken in small amounts (3 to 6 ounces). Continue to drink 3 to 6 ounces at 10–15 minute intervals during the game.

Because water is what is being lost from the body, water is needed to replace body fluids. For most people, electrolyte replacement solutions (such as Gatorade®) are not needed during exercise, although they aid recovery after play is over.

If proper fluid levels are maintained by drinking water before, during, and after playing, overheating should not be a problem. Moreover, you will not fatigue as quickly during the game as a result of water loss and dehydration. For your own safety, begin each game of racquetball with a drink of water!

Points to Remember

→ Before playing, prepare your body with a good warm-up. The warm-up should relax your body, increase your heart rate, and stretch your muscles.

→ Relax by sitting comfortably for a few minutes before beginning any activity. Breathe easily, and exhale completely.

→ Increase your heart rate by stair-stepping, cycling, running in place, or rope-skipping.

→ Stretch when the muscles are warm. Begin with exercises for the upper body, and work down. Stretch the large muscles first, and never bounce during a stretch. Hold all stretches 15 seconds.

→ If muscles become increasingly sore when stretching, STOP. You may have an injury.

→ To be effective, complete the warm-up just before entering the court.

→ Prior to play, focus on the upcoming game.

→ During play, block out extraneous thoughts, and concentrate only on each shot, control your temper and learn from your mistakes.

→ Avoid wearing clothing that traps heat and promotes excessive sweating.

→ Drink 3–6 ounces of cold water every 10–15 minutes during the match.

→ After playing, drink a pint of water for every pound of weight lost.

?????

Self Testing Questions

Answers to Self Testing Questions are located on page 131.

1. There are three phases identified with a proper warm-up, and they are:
   a. relaxation, increase heart rate, stretching.
   b. relaxation, decrease heart rate, stretching.
   c. psyching up, increase heart rate, stretching.
   d. psyching up, relaxation, stretching.

2. When stretching,
   a. begin at the head and work down the body.
   b. stretch small muscles first and then the large muscles.
   c. bounce on stretches.
   d. force a stretch to ensure a good stretch.

3. Stretching assists a player before beginning competition to
   a. relieve muscle contraction and prevent tight muscles.
   b. avoid fatiguing muscles.
   c. loosen the joints and muscles to prepare for fast movements.
   d. relieve muscle contraction, prevent tight muscles, and avoid muscle fatigue.

4. Mental readiness requires a player to
   a. be mentally tough.
   b. concentrate on playing the game.
   c. block outside influences.
   d. be mentally tough, concentrate on the game, and block outside influences.

5. When playing more than 30 minutes during a game, a player should consume
   a. 3 ounces of liquid every 5–10 minutes.
   b. 3–6 ounces of liquid every 10–15 minutes.
   c. 3–6 ounces of liquid every 15–20 minutes.
   d. 6–9 ounces of liquid every 30 minutes.

6. Describe an upper body stretch activity and identify the area stretched.

   _____

   _____

   _____

   _____

   _____

   _____

   _____

7. Describe a lower body stretch activity and identify the area stretched.

   _____

   _____

   _____

   _____

   _____

   _____

   _____

8. If, when stretching, the muscle becomes sore you should
   a. stop stretching.
   b. ease off.
   c. increase effort.
   d. stop for a 30–60 second period and then stretch again.

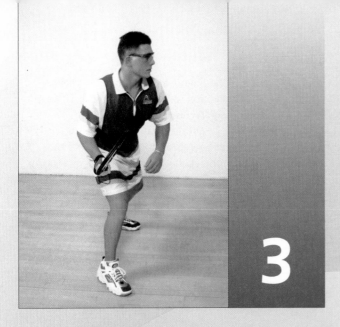

3

Preliminaries to the Strokes in Racquetball

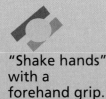

"Shake hands" with a forehand grip.

Being properly prepared to hit the ball is essential to executing offensive and defensive shots correctly. This includes gripping the racquet properly, assuming the set or ready position, and pivoting to either a forehand or backhand hitting position.

Holding the Racquet: the Grips

The power in a racquetball stroke comes from the snap of the wrist that occurs when the ball is contacted. Unless the racquet is gripped in such a way as to maximize this snap, the potential power of a stroke will be lost. Most players use two basic grips during play. A third type of grip may be used in special situations. The first, and easily the most popular, is the **Eastern Forehand**. The Eastern Forehand, as its name implies, is used to hit only shots on the racquet-hand (forehand) side of the body. Its counterpart on the non-racquet-hand side, the Eastern Backhand, will be discussed later.

Eastern Forehand Grip

The easiest way to assume an **Eastern Forehand** grip is merely to hold the racquet on edge so it is perpendicular to the floor and then "shake hands" with the handle (see Figure 3.1). In the shaking-hands position, the first finger and thumb of the racquet hand should form a "V" along the top of the handle, the point of the "V" lying on the midline of the handle's surface (see Figure 3.2).

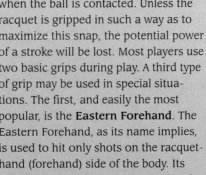

Figure 3.1 Shaking hands with the racquet.

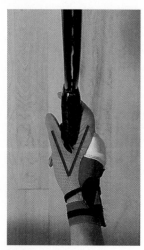

Figure 3.2 Eastern Forehand grip.

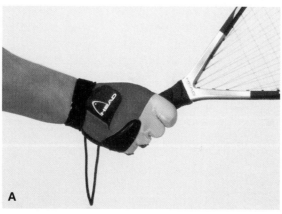

A

Back of hand

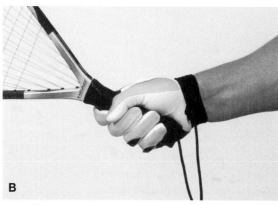

B

Palm of hand

Figure 3.3 Trigger grip.

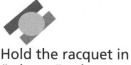

Hold the racquet in a "trigger" grip.

The fingers are spread in a "trigger" position to allow for better wrist snap (see Figure 3.3).

Another way to assume this position is to hold the racquet in the non-racquet hand so the racquet again is on edge. Place your racquet hand with fingers spread on the strings of the racquet so the palm is flat against the racquet face (see Figure 3.4). Slide your racquet hand down the racquet until the end of the handle meets the end of your palm, and wrap your fingers around the handle. Again check to see if the "V" formed by your first finger and thumb is pointed properly along the top bevel (surface) of the handle. Be careful not to grip the racquet so the handle lies perpendicular to your fingers in a "fist" grip, or the wrist snap will be lost (see Figure 3.5). If you turn the racquet over so your palm is pointed toward the ceiling of the court and open your hand, a racquet in the correct position should lie diagonally across the palm (see Figure 3.6). The handle should cover the first knuckle of the first finger and the bottom left side of the palm. The combination of shaking hands, "V" position, and "trigger" finger serve as reminders of an Eastern Forehand grip (see Figure 3.7).

Eastern Backhand Grip

If you use the Eastern Forehand grip for your forehand shots, you must change your grip to hit backhand shots (shots to the non-racquet-hand side). This is because of the way the arm moves

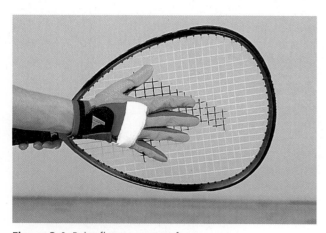

Figure 3.4 Palm flat on racquet face.

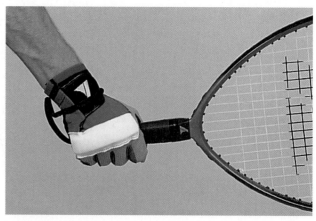

Figure 3.5 Improper grip on racquet, fingers perpendicular to handle.

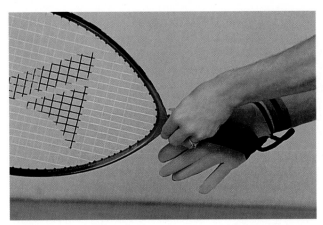

Figure 3.6 Handle of racquet lying diagonally across palm of hand.

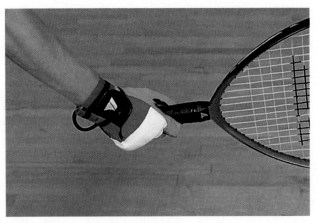

Figure 3.7 Assuming the Eastern Forehand grip.

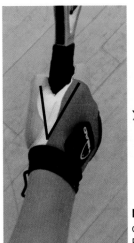

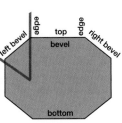

Figure 3.8A Initiation of change to Eastern Backhand grip.

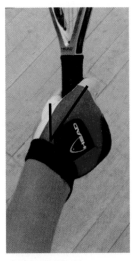

Figure 3.8B The change to the Eastern Backhand grip, and "V".

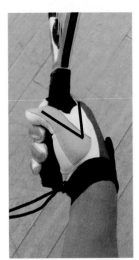

Figure 3.8C Alternative rotation of wrist to hit a backhand shot.

about the elbow. The construction of the elbow joint causes the forearm to move only up and down (flex and extend) when the arm is held straight at your side. When hitting a backhand shot, the racquet arm is pulled across the body and then extended. If the racquet is held with the forehand grip, the racquet head will be turned up when the ball is hit. Thus, shots that should be hit straight into the front wall will be "popped," or hit up toward the ceiling. To hit a level backhand shot, you must change your grip from the Eastern Forehand to the **Eastern Backhand** grip. To find this position on your racquet, assume the

forehand grip just discussed, and hold the racquet on edge. With your non-racquet hand, turn the top of the racquet toward the fingers of your gripping hand so the forefinger-thumb "V" falls on the top left bevel of the racquet. This grip rotates the head of the racquet downward to compensate for the elbow's inability to rotate and allows you to hit a level ball (see Figures 3.8A and 3.8B).

The problem with changing from the forehand to the backhand grip is that it takes *time*. Thus, you will have to recognize immediately when you should hit a backhand shot, to give you as much time as possible to make the switch. A similar problem occurs after taking the backhand shot. The grip must be changed back to the forehand placement. Unfortunately, many players have difficulty changing grips and hitting the ball too! But a player must do something to change the angle of the racquet head.

One alternative solution is to simply rotate the wrist toward the floor when hitting a backhand shot. This turns the racquet head downward and allows a flat shot to be hit (see Figure 3.8C). Returning to the Eastern Forehand grip

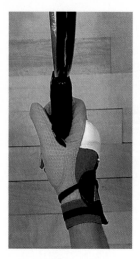

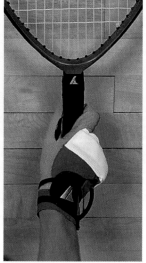

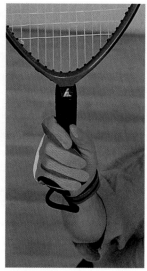

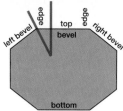

Figure 3.9
Continental grip, and
"V".

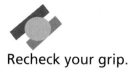

Recheck your grip.

Figure 3.10 Western grip
(front view).

Figure 3.11 Western grip
(back view).

and Backhand. To assume this grip, the racquet must be rotated clockwise one-eighth of a turn from the Eastern Forehand grip. Now the "V" will point to the top left edge of the handle. Thus, with the Continental grip, little or no adjustment must be made for either a forehand or a backhand shot, although the wrist may be slightly rotated clockwise to adjust the face of the racquet during a backhand shot to hit a level ball (see Figure 3.9).

Western Grip

The third grip, called the **Western** grip or "frying pan" grip (see Figures 3.10 and 3.11), is similar to the grip you use on a frying pan handle when you lift the pan off a stove or pick up your racquet off the floor. Some players prefer this grip for overhead forehand shots, but it is not necessary to change to this grip at all if you are not hitting an overhead shot. The Western grip never should be used to hit a forehand or a backhand shot.

After hitting a few balls, always recheck your grip to make sure the racquet has not twisted in your hand. Some players will even mark the "V" placement of the thumb and forefinger with tape on the racquet's top bevel. This helps to guide the correct hand positioning.

takes only a twist of the wrist. The major problem with this method is that it is so easy that new players often *forget* to do it!

Either way of changing the racquet position for a backhand can be effective as long as you use it consistently. Choose one method and practice it all the time.

Continental Grip

A second alternative to changing grips is to avoid using the Eastern Forehand and Backhand grips completely. Instead, use the **Continental** grip. In the Continental grip, the racquet is held in a position midway between the Eastern Forehand

Points to Remember

→ Note the position of the "V" on the racquet handle, and make sure it matches your hand placement.

→ Keep your fingers spread out in a pistol or trigger-finger grip. Don't keep a fist grip on the handle.

→ Change to a backhand grip or compensate for the elbow's movement by rotating the wrist to hit a ball on the non-racquet side. Change back to a forehand grip after taking the shot.

→ Use a Western grip, if desired, to hit overhead shots.

→ All balls can be hit with the Continental grip.

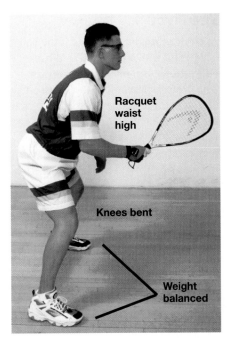

Figure 3.12A Set position (side view).

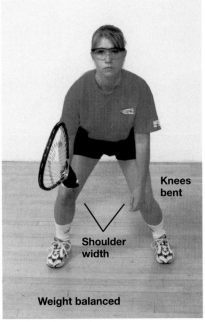

Figure 3.12B Set position (front view).

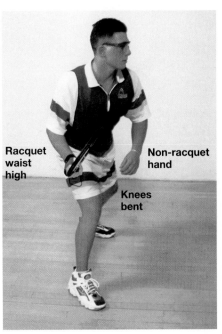

Figure 3.12C Pivot.

Set, Pivot, and Stroke

The Set

The **set** or "ready" position prepares you to hit the ball. Begin each stroke at the set position and return to it following each hit. The set position allows you to move quickly to hit a ball with either your forehand or backhand.

To get in the set position, stand with your feet shoulder-width apart, toes pointing forward, and weight equally balanced on the balls of the feet. Hold the racquet in front of you just below waist height, and use a forehand grip. Your non-racquet hand should be free to provide ease of movement. Knees should be slightly bent and pointed forward. Shoulders, head, and neck are relaxed, with your eyes free to follow the movement of the ball (see Figure 3.12A and 3.12B). Breathing must be deep and regular.

Points to Remember

→ Face the front wall, with toes pointed forward.
→ Balance weight equally on the balls of the feet, placed shoulder-width apart.
→ Hold the racquet with a forehand grip at waist height in front of you.
→ Bend knees, relax head, shoulders, and neck—the body is ready to spring into action.

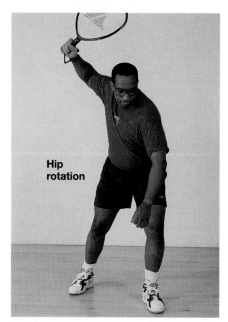

Figure 3.13 Pivot position for forehand stroke.

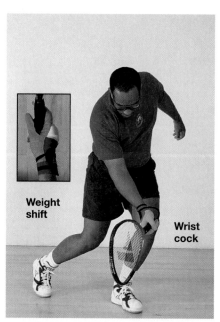

Figure 3.14 Shifting weight into ball from pivot position for forehand stroke.

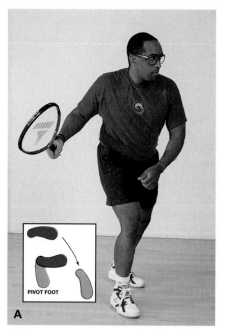

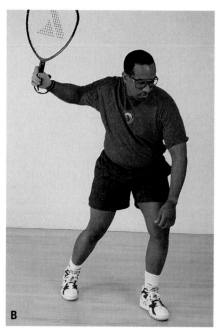

Figure 3.15 Forward pivot for forehand stroke.

The Pivot

As soon as you have decided if the ball is to be hit with a forehand or a backhand stroke, you must **pivot**, or turn your body to prepare for the hit (see Figure 3.12C). The sooner the decision can be made, the better prepared you will be to hit the ball. So decide *quickly*. The importance of the pivot is that it turns the hips sideways to the front wall. This allows the player to step into the ball and add his/her body weight into the power of the stroke (see Figures 3.13 and 3.14).

A baseball batter will take the same position. Except to bunt, the batter will always stand sideways to the pitcher and step into the pitch by shifting his/her weight forward. Thus, the ball can be hit with more force. Similarly, the pivot in racquetball positions you to step into the ball, shift your weight, and increase the power of your stroke. This is especially important for any player who may have weaker arms and wrists.

The pivot may be done by moving either forward or back. In either case, you must shift your weight to one foot to turn and face a side wall. Your free foot will be pulled either forward or behind you to complete the pivot. Your body should finish the pivot with your hips facing a side wall. Whether you pivot and step forward or backward depends on where the ball rebounds and whether you have to move up or back to reach it (see Figures 3.15 and 3.16). Further adjustments in body position can be made by "cross-stepping" or sliding forward or backward. During any pivot motion, your eyes must not lose contact with the ball, and your face should be directed toward the ball.

Points to Remember

→ Decide quickly where the ball is to be hit, and pivot to that side immediately.

→ After the pivot, be sure your body faces a side wall.

→ Move either forward or backward to the ball by cross-stepping or sliding up or back.

→ Keep your eyes and face directed at the ball.

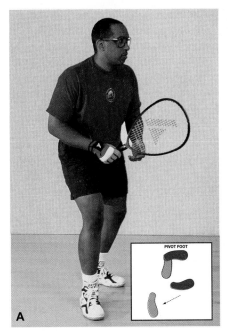

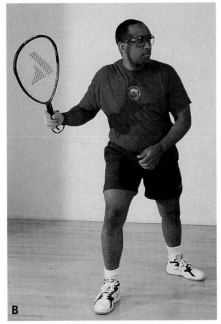

Figure 3.16 Backstep pivot for forehand stroke.

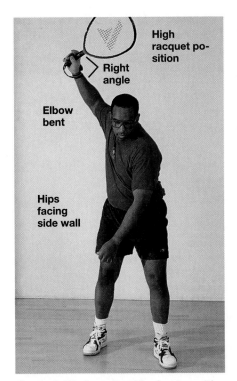

Figure 3.17 Completed backswing with racquet in line between back wall and body.

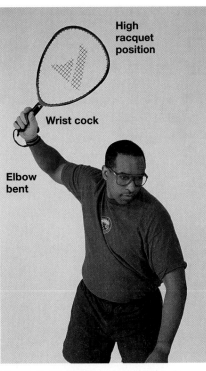

Figure 3.18 Wrist cock on backswing.

Forehand Stroke

The only problem remaining is to hit the ball! **Forehand strokes** will be discussed first, followed by information on backhand strokes. The forehand stroke itself begins as the racquet is carried from the set stance through the position change that results from the pivot.

Backswing

As the body is turned to the side wall, so is the racquet. But the racquet continues to be pulled back so that with the elbow bent, the racquet is in a line between your body and the back wall and held high above the head (see Figure 3.17). This is called the **backswing**. In this position, the racquet is held almost at a right angle to the forearm, which serves to cock the wrist (see Figure 3.18).

Wrist Cock

The **wrist cock** is a critical part of your stroke. The uncocking or snapping of the wrist and racquet at the ball is what generates the speed and power of the stroke. Without cocking the wrist, as in pulling the hammer back on a gun, there would be no way of hitting the ball with explosive force (see Figure 3.18). To be most effective, the snap or uncocking of the wrist must occur when the ball is contacted.

Forward Swing

As you prepare to swing the racquet forward, you first must shift your weight forward (see Figure 3.19). This is done by stepping into the path of the ball with the foot closest to the front wall. During the swing, the elbow must remain close to the side of the body. This position enables the ball to be contacted below waist level and prevents "over-the-shoulder" shots. The racquet hand should lead the racquet through the swing. This position helps to maintain a "cocked" wrist during the swing (see Figure 3.20). The elbow should remain bent until the ball is contacted. At that

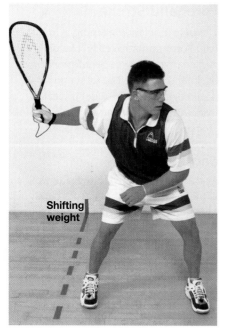

Figure 3.19 Weight shifted forward to contact ball.

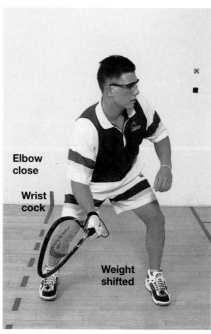

Figure 3.20 Forward swing maintaining wrist cock for forehand stroke.

point, the elbow is extended, the arm straightened, and the racquet head snapped forward to meet the ball. Once the arm is extended, the racquet should be at the same level off the floor as your hand, with the head perpendicular to the floor, or "on edge."

Points to Remember

→ On the backswing, pull the racquet back with elbow bent to a point directly behind you in line with your body and the back wall, racquet held high.
→ To cock the wrist, hold the racquet almost at a right angle to the forearm.
→ On the forward swing, shift weight to your forward foot.
→ Keep the elbow bent on the forward swing; hold the upper arm close to the body.
→ Maintain wrist cock through the swing, with the racquet head trailing the wrist and elbow through the swing.
→ At the point of contact, extend the arm, keep the racquet head perpendicular to the floor at the same level as the hand, and snap the racquet head forward to meet the ball.

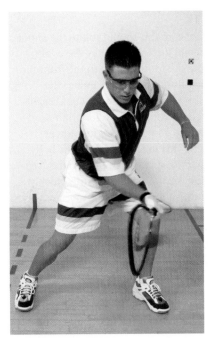

Figure 3.21 Contact point for forehand stroke.

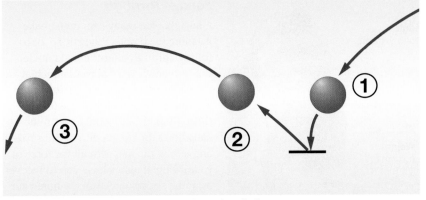

Figure 3.22 Points of contact for a rebounding ball.

Contact

Contact with the ball should be made opposite your forward foot as your weight shifts forward. At the point of impact, the wrist is snapped. In most cases, contact with the ball should be made as close to the ground as possible, with your arm extended. To do this, you must bend your knees to drop your waist and racquet close to the ground. You should not drop the racquet below the level of the hand to hit a low ball, nor should you bend from your waist. Your whole body must lower to ensure that the racquet head remains on edge and moves parallel to the ground (see Figure 3.21).

The ball can be contacted at one of three points during its flight (with reference to Figure 3.22): (1) as it rebounds off the front wall, dropping below your waist toward the floor; (2) after the ball rebounds off the floor and bounces toward your racquet; and (3) after the ball reaches the height of its bounce and is falling back to the floor and below your waist. For experienced players, hitting the ball as it rebounds off the floor (point 2) maintains a fast tempo in the game. The beginning player, however, should wait for the ball to reach the height of its bounce and begin to fall back to the floor for the second time (point 3) before hitting the ball.

Points to Remember

→ Shift your weight onto your forward foot during the forward swing.
→ Hit the ball opposite your forward foot.
→ At the point of impact, snap the wrist and extend the arm.
→ If possible, contact the ball low to the ground by bending your knees and lowering your body to the ball.

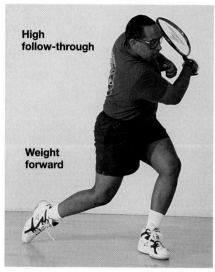

High follow-through

Weight forward

Figure 3.23 Follow-through of forehand stroke.

Follow-Through

A mistake that many beginners make is failing to complete the stroke, or to **follow-through** after the hit is made. Consequently, these players punch at the ball with a shortened stroke and lose the force of their hit. The **follow-through** made after contact with the ball allows for completion of the stroke and hitting the ball with all the force of your swing. It also allows you to recover from the stroke quickly and adjust your stance back to the set position to await your next hit.

In general, a racquetball stroke should end with the racquet swung past the midline of the body and finishing high off the non-racquet side. The follow-through should rotate the shoulders and hips so that they are again facing the front wall, with the front foot acting as a pivot. At the end of the stroke, your weight should be concentrated on your forward foot, but balanced so you do not fall down. During this follow-through, the body should be kept low to the ground (see Figure 3.23). Standing up too quickly will cause the ball to be carried upward with your movement and make it difficult for you to hit low balls. The forehand stroke should follow smoothly in sequential order (see Figure 3.24).

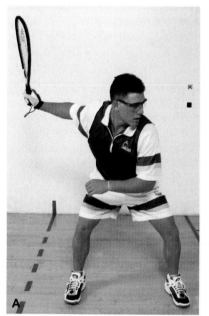

A

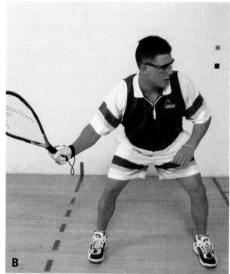

B

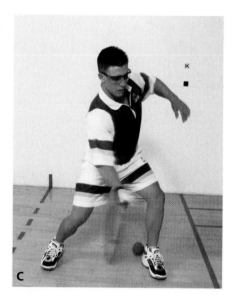

C

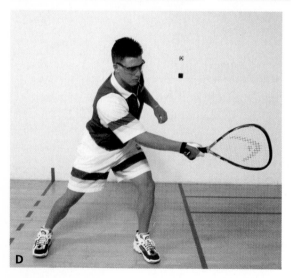

D

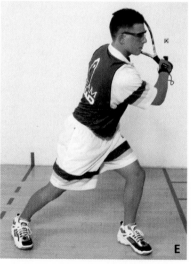

E

Figure 3.24 Forehand drive sequence.

Points to Remember

→ Finish the stroke with the racquet swung past the midline of the body.
→ Stay low, but allow high racquet follow-through.
→ After the ball has been contacted, allow the body to rotate toward the front wall back to the set position following the direction of the arm swing.
→ Don't stand up until the follow-through is complete.

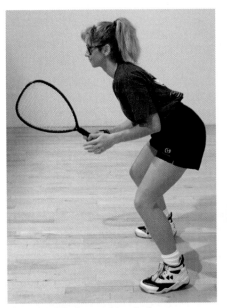

Figure 3.25 Set position before backhand player facing front wall.

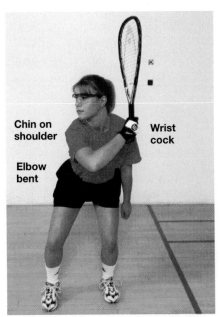

Figure 3.27 Wrist cock for backhand stroke.

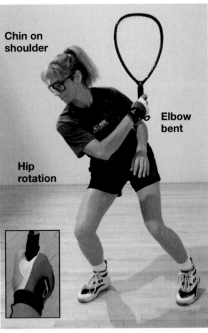

Figure 3.26 Backswing position for backhand stroke.

Backhand Stroke

To hit a **backhand stroke,** use either a backhand grip on the racquet, or turn the racquet face down by rotating the wrist forward. The backhand stroke begins like the forehand stroke from the set position (see Figure 3.25). The pivot, however, results in the player facing the opposite side wall. Again, the pivot can be made by stepping either forward or backward, depending on the position of the ball (see Figure 3.26). After pivoting, the hips should be parallel to the side wall.

Backswing

The backhand stroke is begun by pulling the racquet across the body with the backswing. At the end of the backswing, the racquet is held in line between your shoulder and the back wall with the elbow bent. In this position, the upper body must rotate more than in the forehand stroke for the racquet to be positioned behind the shoulder. When rotated correctly, the chin should almost rest on the shoulder of the racquet arm (see Figure 3.26).

Wrist Cock

The racquet must be held with the **wrist cocked,** as in the forehand stroke. In the cocked position, the racquet is almost at a 90° angle to the forearm (see Figure 3.27).

Forward Swing

As the **forward swing** is begun, the player's weight is shifted to the front foot. The racquet head should trail the elbow and the hand during the forward swing to maintain the cocked position (see Figures 3.28A and 3.28B). The bent elbow should be held close to the body and used as an axis to pivot the racquet around. In error, a beginning player often pulls the elbow (your "wing") out in front of the body toward the front wall (Figure 3.29). When this happens, the racquet head is pulled across the body rather than swung directly at the ball, power is lost, and the ball is rebounded to the side of the court.

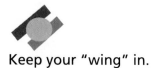

Keep your "wing" in.

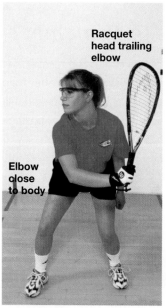

Figure 3.28A Maintain a cocked position.

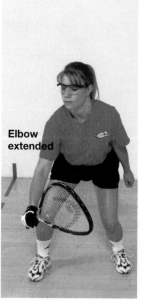

Figure 3.28B Forward swing with racquet trailing hand for backhand stroke.

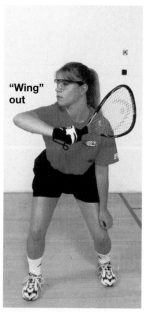

Figure 3.29 Incorrect elbow position.

Points to Remember

→ To change the position of the racquet head to hit the ball, use a backhand grip or rotate your wrist forward.

→ Pivot to the side wall opposite from that turned to with the forehand stroke.

→ Pull the racquet back to a position between the shoulder and the back wall with the elbow bent, racquet held high.

→ Cock the wrist at the end of the backswing.

→ On the forward swing, keep your elbow close to the body and pivot the racquet head around it.

→ Keep the racquet head behind the hand on the forward swing to maintain the wrist cock.

Contact

To contact the ball, your weight should be forward on the front foot. Extend the elbow at the point of contact so the racquet head is now in line with the wrist, elbow, and shoulder. The racquet should contact the ball just opposite the forward foot as low to the ground as possible (see Figure 3.30). When the ball is contacted, the wrist is snapped sharply to bring the racquet in line with the hand and increase the impact on the ball.

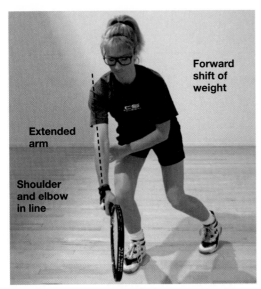

Forward shift of weight

Extended arm

Shoulder and elbow in line

Figure 3.30 Contacting the ball for backhand stroke.

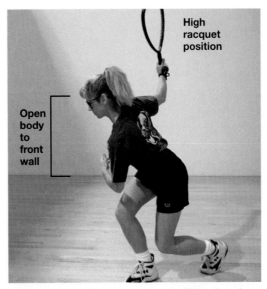

High racquet position

Open body to front wall

Figure 3.31 Follow through on backhand stroke.

Points to Remember

→ Shift your weight forward at contact with the ball.
→ Hit the ball when it is opposite your forward foot and close to the ground.
→ At the point of contact, extend the arm, keeping the elbow close to the body.
→ As the racquet hits the ball, snap the wrist to increase the power in your stroke.

Follow-Through

As with the forehand, the backhand stroke is finished with a **follow-through**. With the follow-through, the chest and hips end up facing the front wall, and the racquet is swung to a point opposite the shoulder of the racquet arm. Without a follow-through, the strength of the swing is lost. Until the stroke is complete, keep your head down to prevent yourself from standing up before the ball leaves the racquet (see Figure 3.31). Otherwise the ball will be lifted up with your movement. Similar to the forehand stroke, the backhand stroke should be executed in one smooth motion (see Figure 3.32).

The success of either a forehand or a backhand stroke depends upon your ability to hit the ball consistently with the same stroking motion. This means that the point of contact with the ball in relation to your body must not vary. The only way to assure this is to *move* on the court so the ball is aligned properly with your stroke. Too many beginning players (and some better ones, too!) are content to hit the ball regardless of where it is, if it is within their reach. This tactic results in many unorthodox strokes in an attempt to hit the ball. Since most of these shots have never been practiced, these strokes merely rebound the ball back to the front wall rather than being accurately placed. It is the player who is consistently positioned to hit a practiced shot who can make conscious changes in the racquet head angle or force of impact to *direct* the ball away from the opponent's reach. Now *that* is racquetball!

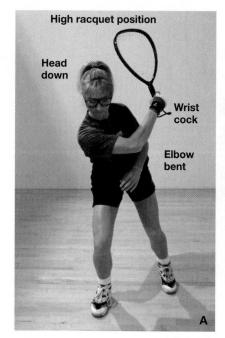

High racquet position

Head down

Wrist cock

Elbow bent

A

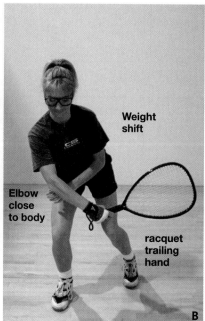

Weight shift

Elbow close to body

racquet trailing hand

B

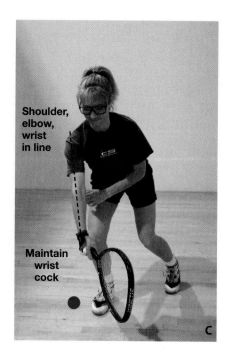

Shoulder, elbow, wrist in line

Maintain wrist cock

C

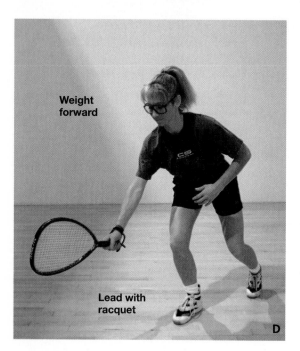

Weight forward

Lead with racquet

D

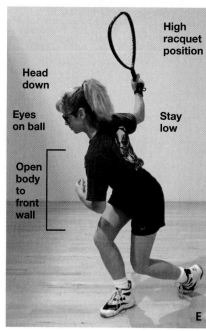

High racquet position

Head down

Eyes on ball

Open body to front wall

Stay low

E

Figure 3.32
Backhand drive sequence.

Points to Remember

→ Finish the stroke with a follow-through so the racquet stops at a point opposite the forward shoulder.

→ Stay low after hitting the ball.

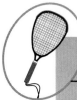

Common Errors and How to Correct Them

1. **I never know where the ball is going.**

You fail to position yourself so the ball is contacted at the same place in relation to your body at all times. Move in the court, and go to where the ball will be. Set yourself up, and hit the ball as you have practiced.

2. **I can't hit the ball hard.**

Check to see if you are following through rather than just punching at the ball and stopping your arm motion.

Make sure your wrist is cocked and you are snapping your wrist at the moment of contact with the ball to increase the impact.

Make sure you are hitting the ball when you shift your weight forward.

3. **The ball always goes up. I can't seem to hit a low ball.**

Check your grip to see if the racquet head is pointed up at contact.

Watch your body position to see if you are standing up before the ball leaves the racquet head. You may be carrying the ball up with you.

Emphasize a low follow-through rather than just punching at the ball.

Let the ball drop lower before you hit it, and keep the racquet perpendicular to the floor.

4. **I miss the ball completely or the ball always hits a side wall first.**

You probably are hitting the ball off your back foot. This area is not in your field of vision, and you lose track of the ball. Hitting the ball from this position also means that your arm has not swung the racquet far enough so the racquet head is parallel to the front wall at contact. Instead, the racquet head is still angled toward a side wall, causing the ball to rebound in that direction.

5. **I hit the ball into the side wall.**

Usually this means you have not changed from the set position to the pivot. Your hips therefore are facing the front wall rather than the side wall. As a result, your stroke comes across the body and directs the ball into the side wall.

If it is a backhand shot, you also may be pulling your elbow in front of your body rather than pivoting around it during the swing.

You could be hitting off your back foot. See answer 4.

6. **I can't hit my backhand with strength and power.**

You are positioning yourself too close to the ball on your backhand side. As a result, you cannot extend your arm and utilize the wrist snap at the point of contact to maximize your power.

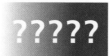

Self Testing Questions

Answers to Self Testing Questions are located on page 131.

1. The Eastern Forehand grip is characterized by
   a. a shake-hands position on the grip with a V formed by the index finger and thumb on top of the grip, and a trigger-finger position on the grip.
   b. a shake-hands position on the top of the grip with a V formed by the finger and thumb on top of the grip, and a grip with the fingers perpendicular to the handle.
   c. a shake-hands position on the grip with a V formed by the index finger and thumb pointed to the racquet-side shoulder, and a trigger-finger position on the grip.
   d. a fist grip with fingers perpendicular to the handle.

2. The position of the V formed by the index finger and thumb when using a Continental grip is positioned
   a. with the V pointed toward the bottom left edge of the handle.
   b. with the V pointed toward the top left edge of the handle.
   c. with the V pointed toward the bottom center of the handle.
   d. with the V pointed toward the top right edge of the handle.

3. The Western grip is used to hit
   a. forehand shots.
   b. backhand shots.
   c. both types of shots.
   d. neither type of shot.

4. The set position requires
   a. racquet positioned waist high and knees bent with weight forward.
   b. racquet positioned waist high and knees bent with weight balanced.
   c. racquet positioned waist high and knees extended with weight balanced.
   d. racquet positioned waist high and knees extended with weight forward.

5. The critical part of a racquetball stroke is
   a. a wrist cock followed by a snap of the wrist at contact.
   b. a firm wrist followed by a sweeping motion at contact.
   c. a firm wrist followed by a snap of the wrist at contact.
   d. a wrist cock followed by a sweeping motion at contact.

6. The follow-through when executing a racquetball basic stroke is characterized by
   a. the racquet and body finishing high with balance on the lead foot.
   b. the racquet finishing high with the body staying low and balance on the lead foot.
   c. the racquet finishing high with the body staying low and balance on the back foot.
   d. the racquet and body finishing high and balance on the back foot.

7. The correction required to eliminate hitting a basic stroke into the side wall first before hitting the front wall is to
   a. pivot from the set position so that your hips are facing the side wall.
   b. make contact with the ball off your lead foot.
   c. neither a or b.
   d. both a and b.

8. When making contact with the ball, the body position should include
   a. stepping away from the ball.
   b. stepping into the ball.
   c. neither a or b.
   d. both a and b.

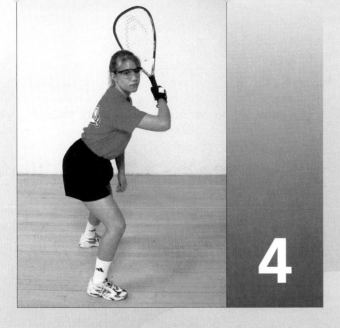

4

Offensive Strokes

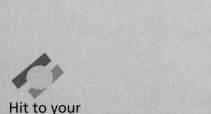

Hit to your
opponent's weak side.

An **offensive shot** is designed to win a point outright by virtue of the skill with which it is hit. Regardless of where your opponent is playing, the well-executed offensive shot should always be a winner. Several basic offensive shots exist. Any offensive shot may be hit with either a forehand or a backhand stroke, and the skilled player can use either stroke with equal effectiveness.

The beginning player will usually choose to hit an offensive shot from the forehand side. This gives credence to the observation of a player having a "weak" side, i.e., one from which an offensive shot is usually not hit (in most cases the backhand). Therefore, a good strategy to follow when playing a *weak-sided* opponent is to hit your offensive shots so that they must be returned with a "weak" side shot (i.e., backhand). With this strategy, if your offensive shot is not perfect, you are usually not setting up an offensive return.

The type of offensive shot you hit is dependent upon your skill with each shot, your position on the court, and in a few instances, your opponent's court position. To hit accurate offensive shots requires hours of practice on the court. Therefore, you should not rely on offensive shots in a game situation until you can hit them consistently in practice.

Kill Shots

A **kill shot** is the ultimate offensive weapon of a racquetball player. By definition, a kill shot is a ball that hits the front wall so low and hard that the rebound to the floor occurs almost simultaneously with the front-wall hit (see Figure 4.1). This rebound makes it virtually impossible for your opponent to return the ball even if he/she is standing in the ball's path.

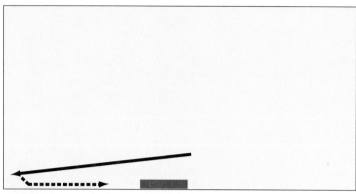

Figure 4.1 Rebound of a kill shot off front wall.

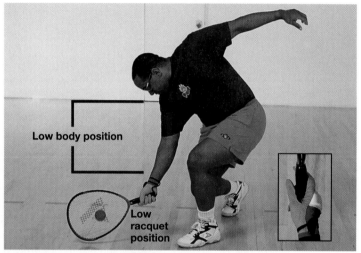

Figure 4.2 Forehand racquet position to hit kill shot.

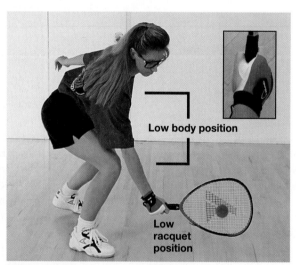

Figure 4.3 Backhand racquet position to hit kill shot.

All kill shots, except the overhead kill, should be hit when the ball is close to the floor. Contact with the ball must be made by bending your knees to drop your waist and racquet arm close to the floor. Ideally, the ball should be struck when it is positioned between your bent knee and the top of your foot (see Figures 4.2 and 4.3). The shot is then made with a normal forehand or backhand motion, with emphasis on generating power in the hit by stepping into the ball and using a good wrist snap (see Figures 4.4 and 4.5). The harder the ball is hit, the farther away from the front wall a kill shot can be successfully made. Most beginners, however, because of their weaker stroke, should concentrate on hitting kill shots from a mid-court position or just behind the short line.

The critical factor in hitting a good kill shot is keeping the racquet perpendicular to the floor and the swing parallel to the floor to ensure hitting a flat or level ball. A level hit will rebound off the front wall at or below the height that it hits into the wall. Thus, a low, level ball hit to the front wall has the greatest potential for achieving the desired kill shot effect (see Figure 4.6).

Front Wall–Straight-In Kill Shot

A **front wall–straight-in kill** shot hits the front wall first and rebounds toward the back wall without touching a side wall. This shot can be hit from anyplace in the court and at any time during play, but it is most effective if your opponent is (A) next to, or (B) behind you in the court (see Figure 4.7). Ideally, this kill shot should be directed toward the half of the front wall farthest away from the opposing player. Since the ball follows a straight path to the front wall, the racquet face must be parallel to this surface when it strikes the ball. In addition, keeping the swing level to the floor will ensure that the ball is hit low to the front wall.

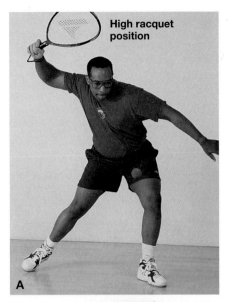

High racquet position

A

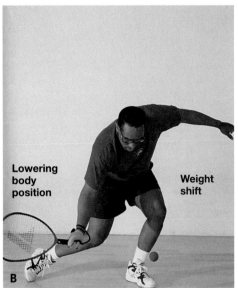

Lowering body position

Weight shift

B

Figure 4.4
Forehand kill shot sequence.

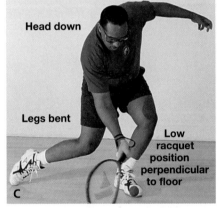

Head down

Legs bent

Low racquet position perpendicular to floor

C

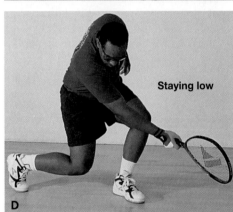

Staying low

D

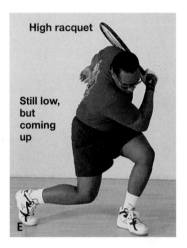

High racquet

Still low, but coming up

E

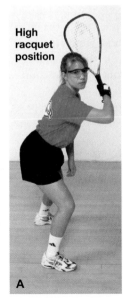

High racquet position

A

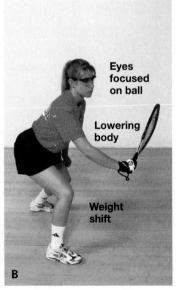

Eyes focused on ball

Lowering body

Weight shift

B

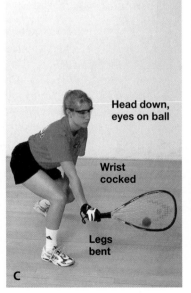

Head down, eyes on ball

Wrist cocked

Legs bent

C

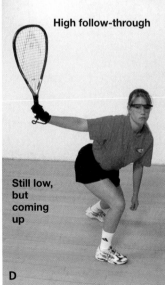

High follow-through

Still low, but coming up

D

Figure 4.5 Backhand kill shot sequence.

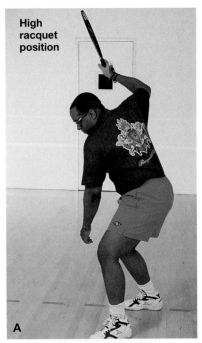
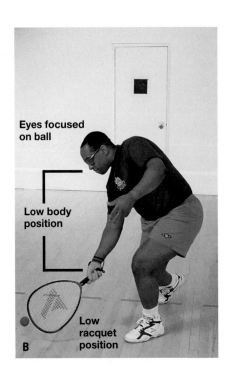
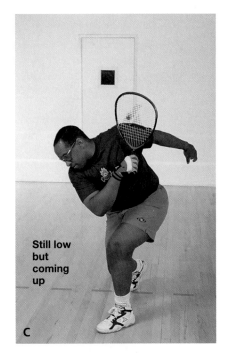

Figure 4.6 Forehand kill shot.

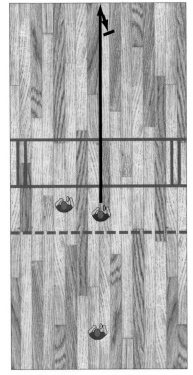

Figure 4.7 Front wall–straight-in kill shot.

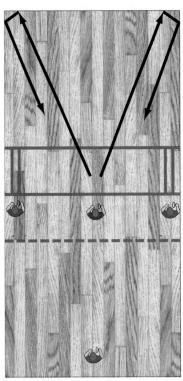

Figure 4.8 Front wall–side wall kill (corner).

Front Wall–Side Wall Kill (Corner)

As shown in Figure 4.8, if the opponent is (A) close to a side wall, or (B) in the back court, a **corner kill** may be used. In this shot, the racquet is held so that at the point of contact, the ball is aimed at a corner of the front wall (see Figure 4.9). As a result, the ball will hit the front wall close to a front wall–side wall crotch and quickly rebound to the nearest side wall. Depending upon the angle at which the ball is hit, the ball may bounce toward a front- or a mid-court position. The success of this shot depends on your opponent's court position and how accurately you can hit the ball. If the ball is not hit low as a kill shot should be, or if the opponent is not far enough in the back court or toward a side wall, the shot will be a setup for an easy return to the front wall. One way to adjust for a quick-reacting opponent who covers the court well is to hit the corner kill at a sharper angle closer to the corner so that the ball rebounds toward the front-court position.

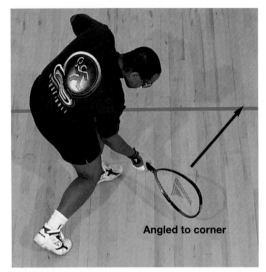

Figure 4.9 Racquet head angled to front corner for kill shot.

Angled to corner

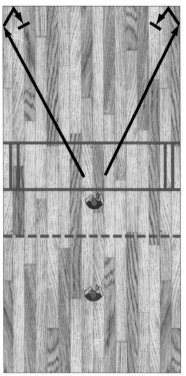

Figure 4.10 Side wall–front wall kill (pinch).

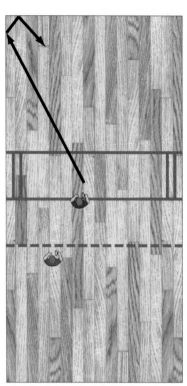

Figure 4.11 Pinch kill hit away from opponent.

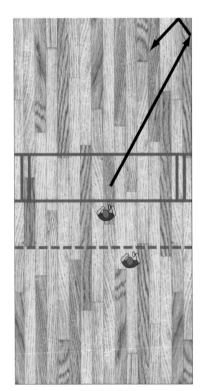

Figure 4.12 Pinch kill hit to opponent's backhand.

Side Wall–Front Wall Kill (Pinch)

The **pinch kill** shot hits one side wall before rebounding into the front wall. An advantage of hitting the pinch kill rather than the corner kill is simply the placement of the rebounding ball. Where the corner kill is more likely to rebound close to a mid-court position, the pinch kill rebounds tightly into the front court (see Figure 4.10). However, to be most effective with the pinch kill, the opponent should be next to or behind you in the court.

Whether the shot is directed to the left or the right front corner depends partly on your position in the court, but more importantly on your opponent's position. Ideally, you should always hit the ball so that the rebound off the front wall is traveling away from the opponent (see Figure 4.11). If this can't be done, at least hit the ball so that it rebounds toward the opponent's weak side. A shot to the weak side, even if not perfectly hit, should not result in an offensive return (see Figures 4.12 and 4.13).

To hit a pinch kill (as with the corner kill), the racquet face upon contact with the ball must be angled to the side wall rather than held parallel to the front wall. The ball must be contacted close to the ground. To do this, bend your knees, drop your waist, and extend your racquet arm down (see Figure 4.9). In all other respects, the technique for hitting this kill shot is similar to that for a forehand or backhand stroke (see Figures 3.24, page 32 and 3.32, page 36).

The pinch kill is ideal for the beginning player because he/she can make a mistake in hitting this shot and still score a point. Since the rebound is to a front-court position, even a ball hit too high or one that rebounds off the floor may be impossible for your opponent to reach as long as he/she is in the back court.

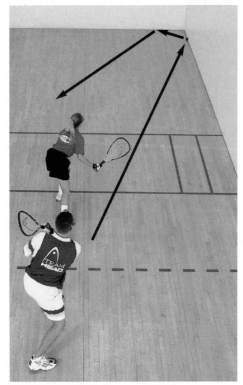

Figure 4.13 Pinch kill hit to opponent's weak side.

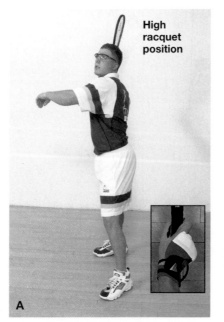

High racquet position

A

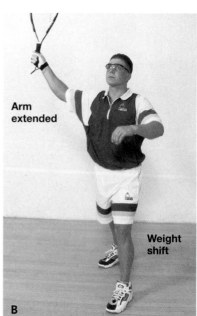

Arm extended

Weight shift

B

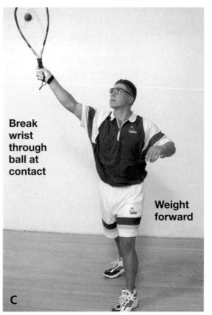

Break wrist through ball at contact

Weight forward

C

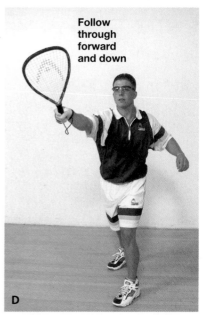

Follow through forward and down

D

Figure 4.14 Forehand overhead kill shot sequence.

Overhead Kill

The **overhead kill** shot is popular with beginning players but falls out of favor as the player develops other offensive weapons. The object of the overhead kill is the same as for any kill shot, but the stroking technique is different. This kill shot is hit from a ball that is above shoulder level rather than close to the ground. It is hit from the forehand side with a motion similar to a tennis serve (see Figure 4.14). The stroke is begun by pulling the racquet back as if to hit a forehand stroke. As the forward swing is begun, however, the racquet is lifted in a circular motion as if you were going to throw it to the front wall. The chest and hips are rotated to face the front wall as you step forward to hit the ball. The ball is contacted just in front of the forward foot with an extended arm.

At contact, the face of the racquet should be angled slightly down to the

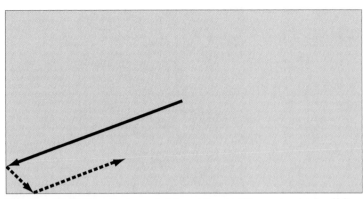

Figure 4.15 Rebound of poorly hit overhead kill bouncing high off floor.

With an overhead kill shot, "throw" the racquet at the ball.

front wall. To assume this position, a Western grip is preferred over any other forehand grip in order to point the face of the racquet to the front wall. To maximize the power of the stroke, the ball always should be hit with the arm in an extended position with a downward wrist snap. Complete the stroke with a follow-through, bringing the racquet through the ball toward the target.

Ideally, the ball should be directed low into the front corner of the court. To have the best chance of success, the overhead kill should hit a side wall as well as the front wall to deaden the rebound of the ball. Otherwise, if not hit perfectly, the ball will rebound high into the air at the same angle at which it hit

the wall (see Figure 4.15). The high bounce gives even a slow opponent adequate time to position himself/herself for the return. Consequently, the overhead kill is considered a "low-percentage" shot because it is hard to score a point off a ball that is not hit perfectly.

Beginning players are advised to be patient and wait for the ball to drop below waist level rather than hit an overhead kill. Then, a corner or pinch kill can be hit. Both of these kill shots are more difficult to return than the overhead kill, even if they are hit incorrectly.

Points to Remember

→ To hit an effective kill shot, wait for the ball to fall low to the floor—at least below your knee.
→ To reach the ball, pivot, bend your knees, and drop your waist to lower your racquet arm toward the ground.
→ To hit a straight-in kill shot, keep your racquet face perpendicular to the floor and parallel to the front wall. Swing level with the floor using a good wrist snap.
→ To direct a kill shot to a front corner, angle your racquet face to the corner that you wish to hit.
→ Try to angle your kill shot away from your opponent's court position or hit to his/her weak side to ensure a successful shot.

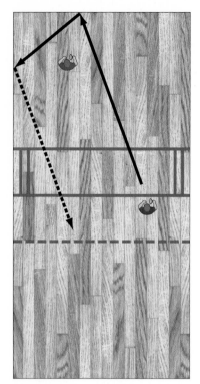

Figure 4.16 Passing shot hit when opponent is caught in front court.

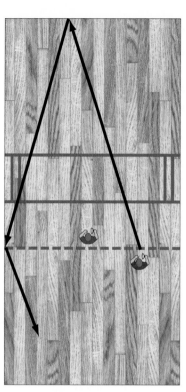

Figure 4.17 Passing shot hit when opponent is positioned in center court.

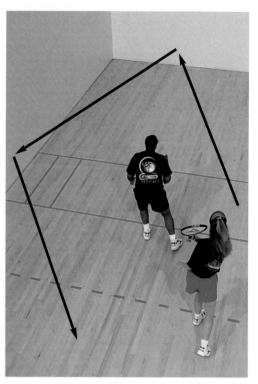

Figure 4.18 Passing shot hitting side wall at same distance from front wall that opponent is standing.

Passing Shots

A **passing shot**, unlike the kill shot, requires no new techniques to master. Its effectiveness depends only on your opponent's court position and your ability to place the ball. The passing shot, as its name implies, is a ball that literally goes past the opponent. Therefore, it is most advantageous to hit when the opposing player is in the front-, mid-, or center-court areas. In this way, the ball can go past the opponent and beat him/her into the back court (see Figures 4.16 and 4.17).

If hit low off the front wall, a passing shot will die in the back court and not rebound into a center-court position. Without rebounding hard off the back wall, the ball in essence is out-of-play, except to a heroic effort. At the very least, if the ball is returned, it usually will be a desperation shot that you can return for a winner, or it will push your opponent to use up his/her energy reserves.

The most critical error beginning players make when using a passing shot

is to hit the ball with too much force. As a result, instead of dying in the back court, the ball rebounds off the back wall into play and negates the advantage the passing shot offers.

The passing shot can be hit with a forehand, a backhand, or an overhead stroke. The ball should be directed to hit the front wall at a point between waist and knee height off the floor. In all cases, however, the lower the rebound off the front wall, the less chance that a return will be made. The ball can be hit directly to a back corner, or it can be angled to rebound from the front wall to contact a side wall on the way to the back court. If the ball is angled toward a side wall, it should hit at the same distance or farther from the front wall as your opponent is standing (see Figure 4.18). This will not only help to slow the movement of the ball into the back court, but also discourage your opponent from trying to hit the ball as it rebounds off the front wall, because it will be out of reach. If the ball hits the

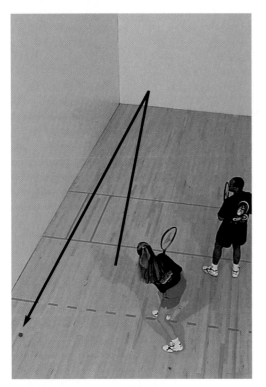

Figure 4.19 Down-the-line pass.

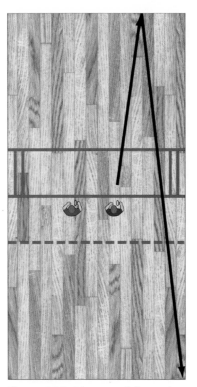

Figure 4.20 Diagram of down-the-line pass.

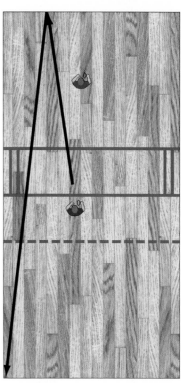

Figure 4.21 Passing shot when opponent is in front court, to weak side.

Ideally, "pass" your opponent on the weak side.

side wall in front of your opponent's court position, it will pass through the center court and allow your opponent to make a play on the ball.

Two types of passing shots are common: the down-the-line pass and the cross-court pass.

Down-The-Line Pass

The **down-the-line pass** could really be called the down-the-wall (wallpaper) pass. This ball is hit so it travels in a line along the side wall, 1 to 3 feet from it and below waist level. As stated before, hitting the ball too hard will cause a strong rebound off the back wall and possibly allow a return to be made. This passing shot ideally is hit when you are between your opponent and the side wall down which you are hitting, or when the opposing player is caught off-guard in a front-court position (see Figures 4.19, 4.20, and 4.21). In either case, hit the ball toward the side wall that is the farthest distance from your opponent. If he/she is playing a center-court position, hit to the backhand side. Use a

forehand stroke to hit down-the-line passing shots to the forehand side of the court and a backhand stroke for balls directed to the backhand side.

Cross-Court Pass

The **cross-court pass** moves the ball from one side of the court to the other in order to pass the opponent. It does this by following the path of a "V" across the court (see Figures 4.22 and 4.23). Depending upon where you are positioned in the court, the ball will rebound off the front wall close to its center. You must experiment with the exact placement of the ball as you hit from different court positions. What will always be true is that the ball will rebound from the front wall at an angle equal to the angle of impact. To prevent the opponent from hitting the rebound off the front wall, this angle must be great enough to avoid the opponent's reach.

As with a down-the-line pass, the cross-court shot may be hit with a forehand, backhand, or overhead stroke.

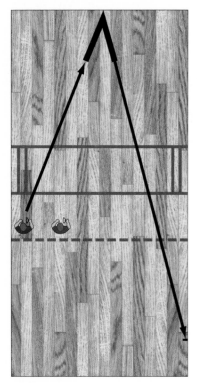

Figure 4.22 Cross-court passing shot with opponent close to side wall.

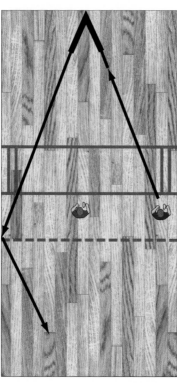

Figure 4.23 Cross-court passing shot with opponent in center court.

It is ideally used when your opponent is forward on your side of the court, is in a center-court position, or is positioned closer to a side wall. One advantage of the cross-court passing shot is that it can be hit from anyplace on the court, including the back court, as the success of the shot depends on your opponent's court position. It is an easy shot to learn and win with because most right-handed players can use their stronger forehands to hit cross-court passing shots to their opponents' weaker backhands.

As with a down-the-line pass, a ball that rebounds low into the back court has the greatest chance of success. This ball also may hit a side wall before rebounding into the back-court area (see Figure 4.23). As stated earlier, however, care must be taken to ensure that the ball does not rebound through a center-court position or in front of the opponent. Hitting a side wall also will help to slow the speed of the ball on the court, allowing you to hit the ball with more force and still have a successful passing shot.

Because a wide margin of error exists with how hard and at what angle the ball should be hit, successful cross-court passing shots can be made by even the beginning player.

Points to Remember

→ A passing shot can be hit with any stroke. Its success is dependent upon your opponent's court position.

→ A passing shot should not be used when your opponent is in a back-court position.

→ A passing shot can be hit cross-court or down-the-line from anyplace on the court.

→ As long as the ball goes into the back court, the lower the passing shot rebounds off the front wall, the greater its chance of being a winning shot.

→ The passing shot may hit a side wall after rebounding from the front wall, but it should not be angled to hit in front of the opponent or to go through the center-court area.

→ Hitting the passing shot too hard will cause the ball to rebound off the back wall into play.

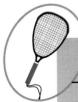

Common Errors and How to Correct Them

1. **My kill shots always hit the floor before they reach the front wall.**

You probably have angled the racquet face down at the point of impact with the ball, driving the ball into the floor. Concentrate on keeping your racquet face perpendicular to the floor and the stroke parallel to the floor.

2. **My kill shots are never low enough to the front wall.**

Be patient and wait for the ball to drop closer to the floor before hitting it. This means that you will have to bend your knees and lower your waist to drop your racquet to the ball. Try to make contact with the ball just off the tops of your shoes. If this does not help, you may be scooping at the ball with the racquet and hitting it on the upswing, which lifts the ball to the front wall higher than you want it to hit. A level swing with the floor will correct this problem.

3. **I hit my cross-court shots right back to my opponent because the ball bounces off a side wall into the center court.**

Take some angle off your hit and aim more for the center of the front wall.

4. **My down-the-line passing shot always hits the side wall.**

The racquet head is not parallel to the front wall when you contact the ball, but instead is angled toward the side wall you are hitting. Snap your wrist and swing through the ball. Also, check to make sure you are contacting the ball off your forward foot. Contacting the ball off your back foot can cause the ball to rebound into the side wall after hitting the front wall.

5. **My overhead kill shot hits (a) the floor first or (b) too high off the front wall.**

When the floor is hit first, the ball is hit either when it is too far in front of you or when your wrist is bent too much, causing the racquet head to be angled to the floor. Check the position of your body relative to the ball when you hit the overhead, and hold the racquet so it appears to be an extension of your arm.

Hitting the ball too high off the front wall usually results from hitting the ball too far behind your front foot or even over your head, which prevents you from angling the hit downward. Again, check the position of the ball when you make contact, and be sure that the contact point is in front of your forward foot.

6. **My passing shots always rebound off the back wall into a center-court position.**

Take some of the force off your stroke, and hit the ball lower off the front wall to ensure a shorter rebound from the back. If this does not help, try to hit a side wall to deaden the ball's movement.

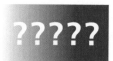

Self Testing Questions

Answers to Self Testing Questions are located on page 131.

1. A kill shot can best be described as the ultimate offensive weapon that strikes the

   a. front wall low and hard with the rebound of the ball contacting the floor almost at the same time as the front wall.

   b. front wall at knee level or lower and rebounds low off the wall.

   c. front wall low and hard with the ball rebounding deep to the back wall.

   d. front wall at knee level or lower and rebounds to the back wall.

2. The critical factor in hitting a kill shot is

   a. keeping the racquet perpendicular to the floor and the swing with racquet face closed.

   b. keeping the racquet perpendicular to the floor and the swing parallel to the floor.

   c. keeping the racquet at a 45-degree angle to the floor and the swing with racquet face closed.

   d. keeping the racquet at a 45-degree angle to the floor and the swing parallel to the floor.

3. The corner kill combination is

   a. front wall, side wall.

   b. side wall, front wall.

4. The pinch kill combination is

   a. front wall, side wall.

   b. side wall, front wall.

   c. both a and b.

5. An overhead kill shot is

   a. contacted from a high racquet position and the ball strikes the front wall low with a high bounce.

   b. contacted with a high racquet position and the ball strikes the front wall low with the ball contacting the front wall and the floor almost at the same time.

   c. contacted from a high racquet position and the ball strikes the side wall and front wall corner.

   d. contacted from a low racquet position and the ball strikes the front wall and side wall corner.

6. A down-the-line passing shot is hit

   a. down the side wall 1–3 feet from the wall and above waist level.

   b. down the side wall 1–3 feet from the wall and below waist level.

   c. down the side wall grazing the wall at below waist level.

   d. down the side wall grazing the wall at above waist level.

7. A cross-court passing shot

   a. is hit low, striking the front wall and rebounding in the path of a V.

   b. is hit high, striking the front wall and rebounding in the path of a V.

   c. is hit low, striking the front and side walls in the path of a V.

   d. is hit high, striking the front and side walls in the path of a V.

8. Cross-court passing shots that strike the front and side wall returning to your opponent can be corrected by

   a. hitting with more angle.

   b. hitting with less angle.

   c. aiming more to the center of the front wall.

   d. none of the above.

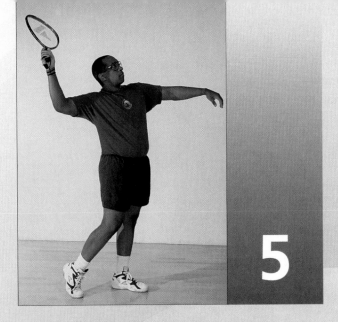

5

Defensive Strokes

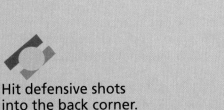

Hit defensive shots
into the back corner.

Rather than scoring a point, the purpose of a **defensive shot** is to *prevent* your opponent from hitting a winning shot. This goal can be achieved only if the ball rebounds high off the front wall, preventing a kill-shot return, or rebounds to a court position that does not favor an offensive return. The best defensive shot is hit in such a way as to have the ball rebound from the front wall high into the back court and close to the side wall. Several strokes accomplish this purpose, at least one of which should immediately become part of your repertoire of shots.

Ceiling–Front Wall Shots

A **ceiling–front wall shot** can be hit with either a forehand or a backhand from any part of the court. A ceiling –front wall shot hits the ceiling before it hits the front wall. Upon contact with the ceiling, the ball rebounds to the front wall close to the ceiling–front wall crotch and then is directed downward to bounce on the floor, hitting in front of the service zone before bouncing into the back-court area (see Figure 5.1).

To hit this shot properly, the ball should be directed to hit the ceiling approximately 2 to 3 feet from the

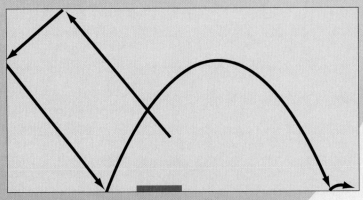

Figure 5.1 Ceiling–front wall defensive shot.

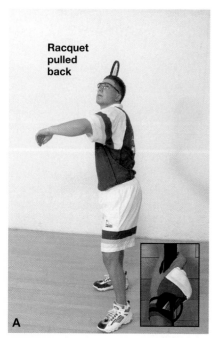

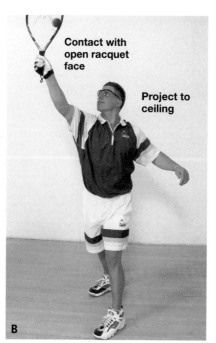

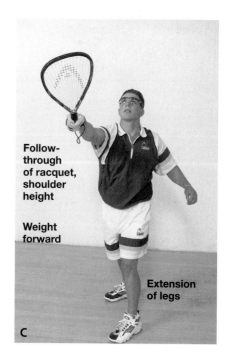

Figure 5.2 Forehand overhead ceiling shot sequence.

ceiling–front wall crotch. The advantage of a ceiling–front wall shot is that it can be an effective defensive shot even if your opponent is near the center court. This is because the rebound of the ball off the floor will carry it high over the head of the opponent and, hopefully, into the back corner. Because the ball must be returned before striking the floor twice, your opponent must hit the ball from this corner position before the ball touches the floor again. Thus, this court position makes it difficult to hit an offensive shot because of the ball's proximity to the walls.

More important, this is an easy shot to learn because the harder you hit the ceiling–front wall shot, the higher the height of the bounce off the floor, and the ball will still land in the back court. Thus, this is not a shot that requires finesse to hit effectively and can be used successfully with relatively little practice.

The ceiling–front wall shot is used most typically on a ball that can be hit with an overhead stroke, either on the forehand (Figure 5.2) or backhand (Figure 5.3) side. For this reason, an overhead ceiling–front wall shot is similar in technique to an overhead kill shot (see Chapter 4). However, unlike

the kill shot, contact with the ball can be made just off the forward foot, with the hips and chest facing the front wall and the arm extended. When hitting a ceiling shot, many players prefer a Western grip, as it opens the face of the racquet to the ceiling.

The difference between the ceiling shot and the offensive kill return is the angle of the racquet face when it contacts the ball. With the ceiling shot, the face must be angled toward the ceiling. To do this, the wrist cannot be snapped from its laid-back position (Figure 5.4) on the forward swing. This will keep the racquet directed upward. The stroke should finish with a follow-through to ensure hitting the ball with power.

A ceiling–front wall shot also can be hit from a ball that has dropped below waist level. For this shot, the stroke begins like any other forehand or backhand stroke. The pivot to the side wall is followed by the backswing with the wrist cocked. As the forward swing is begun, however, the racquet head must be turned back, or "opened," toward the ceiling (see Figure 5.5). This racquet face position directs the ball toward the ceiling. Although this can be an effective shot for novice players, more advanced players usually will take advantage of

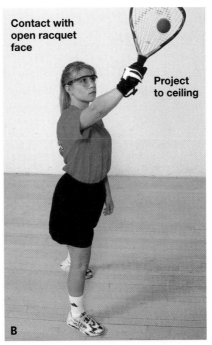
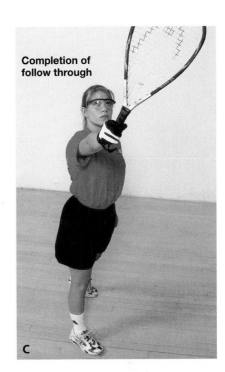

Figure 5.3 Backhand overhead ceiling shot sequence.

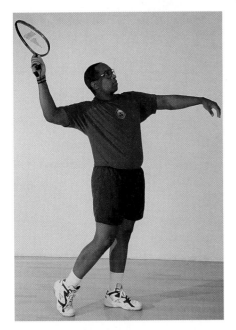

Figure 5.4 Laid-back racquet for forehand overhead ceiling shot.

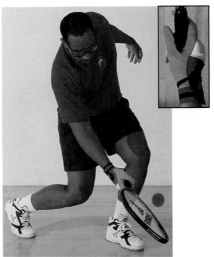

Figure 5.5 Open racquet for ceiling shot.

the low position of the ball in relation to the front wall to try to hit an offensive return rather than a ceiling–front wall return.

To ensure the most difficult return possible, the ceiling–front wall shot should be directed to run along a side wall before it bounces into the back corner. If, in addition, the ball is directed to your opponent's backhand side, this defensive shot may not only result in a

weak return, but possibly no return at all. Thus, this defensive shot actually may score a point for you.

Because a ceiling–front wall shot can be hit from any part of the court, it should be practiced from all court positions. If you are standing to one side of center, you can hit the shot down the closest wall (wallpaper shot) or hit cross-court to the opposite corner. The cross-court ceiling shot requires more power in the stroke because of the longer diagonal court distance to be covered as well as the need for accurate placement. If the ball is not hit at a sharp angle, the rebound forward will be away from the side wall and will provide for easy stroking room. A similar problem exists with a ceiling shot hit down-the-line if it does not hug the wall.

Thus, although the ceiling shot is one of the easiest defensive strokes to learn, if the player does not take time to practice placement, he/she cannot achieve the true advantage of the shot. If the ceiling shot is hit well, it can be used to (1) keep the ball in play, (2) move your opponent to a back-court position, and (3) force a return that is not an offensive shot.

Points to Remember

→ When the ball hits the racquet, direct the angle of the racquet head to the spot on the front wall or ceiling that you want the ball to hit.

→ To hit a ceiling shot from a ball below waist level, open the racquet face.

→ With ceiling shots hit with an overhead stroke, contact the ball just off the forward foot with an extended arm.

→ For the best advantage, angle ceiling shots so they rebound into a back corner, preferably to your opponent's backhand.

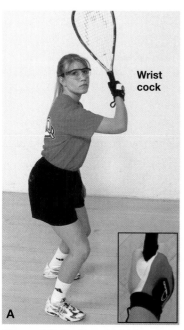

Wrist cock

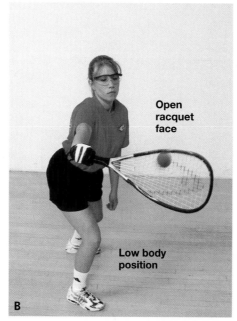

Open racquet face

Low body position

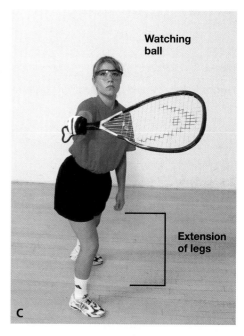

Watching ball

Extension of legs

Figure 5.6 Backhand lob shot sequence.

NEVER hit a lob into the middle of the court.

Lob Shot

A **lob** shot is not played as often in competitive racquetball as other defensive shots. This is because of the popularity of the composite/graphite racquets and pressurized balls. The **lob** is a shot that requires finesse and placement, not the power and strength for which this equipment was designed. Therefore, players who choose a fast-moving, power game often do not have the finesse necessary to hit a lob return.

A lob is used to hit a ball below head level with a technique similar to a ceiling shot. Both shots, whether hit with a forehand or a backhand stroke,

require an open racquet face. Contact with the ball should be made inside the forward foot with an extended arm. Although not much force is required to hit this ball properly, the ball should be struck with your weight shifted toward the front wall. Finish the stroke with a follow-through high over your head. This arm motion and the racquet face angle serve to lift the ball (see Figure 5.6).

Like the ceiling shot, the lob is returned high to the front wall, approximately 6 to 8 feet from the ceiling. The lob shot differs from the ceiling shot in

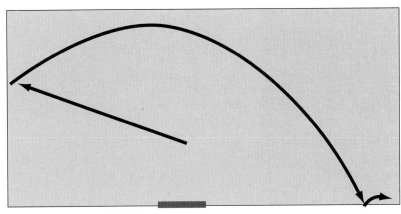

Figure 5.7 Proper lob defensive shot.

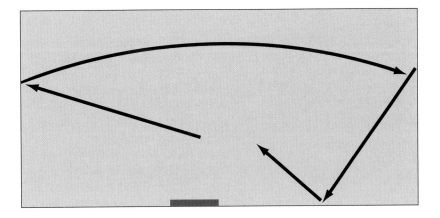

Figure 5.8 Lob shot rebounding into center court off back wall.

on the court, yet forces your opponent into the disadvantage of a back-corner return (see Figure 5.7).

Similar to the ceiling shot, a lob may be hit down-the-line (along the wall) or cross-court. If the lob is hit down-the-line, it is preferable to use a backhand shot toward the non-racquet side wall and a forehand shot to the racquet-hand side wall for more control.

A cross-court lob may be hit with either stroke. The purpose of both shots is to place the ball in a back-court position to prevent an offensive return. Thus, the lob presents many of the same problems to your opponent as the ceiling shot does. The reason why it is not hit more often is because it is a difficult shot to hit correctly. The ball does not rebound from the ceiling on the way to the back court. If hit too hard, the ball will merely rebound off the back wall into a center-court position (see Figure 5.8). Thus, the advantage of a back-corner placement is lost. In addition, because the ball moves so slowly, it is easy to hit a strong return unless the lob is placed correctly. To minimize any possible rebound off the back wall, aim the lob so the ball just brushes against a side wall close to the back corner. This "meeting" will slow the ball and deaden its fall to the floor.

For most beginners, the finesse with which this ball must be hit is hard to manage in a game situation where quick movements are necessary. Yet, the lob does offer an interesting variation for the player who can use it, including changing the pace of the game.

that the ball never rebounds to touch the ceiling. Rather, the ball slowly moves along an arc close to the ceiling and high over center court, falling "dead" into a back corner with little or no rebound from the back wall. When hit perfectly, the slow movement of this ball allows you time to reposition yourself

 Points to Remember

→ Pivot the hips and hit the ball with an open racquet face.
→ Hit the ball as hard as you think necessary, then take some force off your swing.
→ Finish the stroke with a follow-through, with the racquet ending up high over your shoulder.
→ To take some power out of your shot, aim the ball to "brush" the side wall close to the back corner.
→ To be more effective, lob only to a back corner.

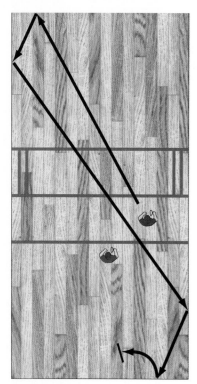

Figure 5.9 High-Z (three-wall) defensive shot.

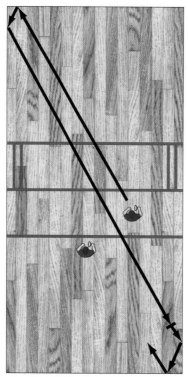

Figure 5.10 High-Z defensive shot hitting floor before back corner.

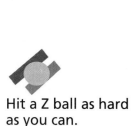

Hit a Z ball as hard as you can.

High-Z Ball or Three-Wall Shot

Like the other defensive shots, the **high Z** or **three-wall shot** is designed to move the opponent into a back corner. The high Z can be hit with either an overhead stroke from a high ball or a forehand or backhand stroke on a low ball return. To ensure proper placement of the ball, the racquet head at contact must again be angled in the direction toward which the ball should travel. This means the racquet face should be slightly open. In all other respects, the high-Z stroke resembles one of the other defensive shots. The overhead stroke is similar to the overhead ceiling shot, and the high Z hit from a lower ball is similar to the lob.

As in other defensive shots, the high Z must be directed to hit high off the front wall. In addition, this shot must hit close to a front wall–side wall crotch (2–3 feet from it). As a result, the ball, after contact with the front wall, rebounds off the nearest side wall and moves diagonally across the court to the back corner. In essence, the movement of the ball describes a "Z" in the court. To follow this path (Figures 5.9 and 5.10), the ball must not hit the ceiling.

The placement of the ball on the front wall is critical to the effectiveness of this shot. If hit too low, the Z ball is an easy setup for your opponent. This is because the ball passes over a center-court position when following the diagonal. A ball hit too low will pass through the center-court area within arm's reach of your opponent. As long as the ball is hit high off the front wall, it will pass high over the center court and force your opponent into a back-court position to return the ball.

Depending upon the strength of the hit, the Z ball may or may not hit a second side wall before touching the floor in the back corner. If hit hard, a second wall will be hit on the opposite side from the first before the ball rebounds to the floor (see Figure 5.9). Thus, the name "three"-wall is often used to identify this shot. In this situation, the ball will "run the corner" by hitting the side wall, the back wall, and then the floor in succession. The ball may also hit the floor before a second wall is touched, deadening its movement as well (see Figure 5.10).

Because the ball covers so much of the court on a Z-ball return, beginning players often do not have a powerful enough stroke to hit the shot well. It is good to practice this shot often and feel confident about hitting it before trying a Z-ball return in a game situation.

Although a Z ball may be hit from anywhere in the court, you should try it from a center-court position if your shot is weak. Stronger players will be effective with a high Z hit even from the back court. Because of the path the ball follows, the Z is best hit to the opposite corner from your court position. Otherwise, the angle off the front wall will not be great enough to cause a rebound along the diagonal.

The Z ball or three-wall shot is effective in causing a weak return,

especially if the ball "runs the corner." In the back corner, there is little room to place a racquet and stroke through the ball unless the timing is perfect and a good wrist snap is used. Therefore, more experienced players often hit this shot not only to force a bad court position but to "handcuff" the opponent as well.

Points to Remember

→ Hit the ball high off the front wall and close to the side wall–front wall crotch.

→ Use a stroke similar to an overhead ceiling shot for a ball over your shoulder, and a lob return for waist-high or lower balls.

→ Hit the ball hard enough to "run the corner" of the back court.

→ Hit the high Z to the corner opposite the side of the court in which you are positioned.

Change the pace with around-the-wall ball.

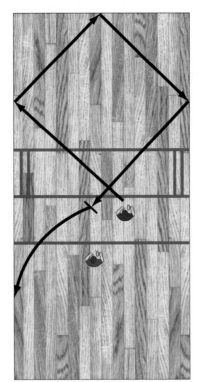

Figure 5.11 Around-the-wall ball.

Around-The-Wall Ball

The around-the-wall ball is a defensive shot that hits three walls before touching the floor. It differs from the high-Z shot in that the ball is first hit high to a side wall. The ball then rebounds to the front wall and finally to the side wall opposite from the initial hit. The closer to the front wall–side wall crotch the ball is aimed, the farther back on the opposite side wall the ball will rebound. Since the purpose of this shot, like other defensive shots, is to force the opponent into a back-court position, hitting close to a front corner is advised. If the ball strikes the first side wall too far from the front, the rebound will merely follow a path back to a center-court position (see Figure 5.11).

The stroke used to hit an around-the-wall ball is the same as for the high Z. This shot must be practiced, however, to ensure that the proper racquet angle is used to hit the ball close to the front corner. Although not used often, the around-the-wall shot is probably most effective against a beginning player who has difficulty determining the rebound angle of the ball, or against any player to change the pace of the game.

Points to Remember

→ Hit the around-the-wall ball with the same technique used for a high-Z ball.

→ For the most effective hit, angle the ball close to the front wall–side wall crotch.

→ Use this ball against beginning players and as a change of pace.

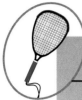

Common Errors and How to Correct Them

1. **My ceiling shots never hit the ceiling.**

If the ball is hit from a position below the waist, you are not hitting with an open racquet face to lift the ball high enough to hit the front wall or ceiling. If you are using an overhead stroke, the ball is probably too far in front of you when you contact it, or your racquet head is not angled toward the ceiling to direct the ball upward.

2. **My ceiling shots hit the ceiling straight over my head.**

For both waist-level and overhead shots, you have angled your racquet too much, and the racquet face is almost parallel to the ceiling. In addition, with the overhead stroke, the ball is probably contacted over your head rather than off your forward foot.

3. **My lob always hits the ceiling.**

You have too much force in your hit or too much angle on the racquet head. Hit the ball softer, and aim for a point lower on the front wall.

4. **My lob always hits the back wall and rebounds to center court.**

Try to angle the hit more into the back corner of the court, then limit the force with which you hit the ball. If the ball does rebound into the court, at least it will be along the wall and still will provide little stroking room.

5. **My high Z does not hit the back-wall corner but goes straight into the back wall.**

Angle your hit into the front wall closer to the front wall–side wall crotch by changing the direction of the racquet head.

6. **My high Z bounces too high off the back wall and gives my opponent an easy return.**

Hit the ball lower to the front wall, or softer and with more of an open racquet face so the ball arcs into the back court.

7. **My high-Z ball always rebounds off the front wall–side wall and bounces at center court, where my opponent returns it.**

Make sure that you are pivoting your hips before you stroke and that you are stepping into the ball. If you rely only on the strength of your arm to hit the ball, the force may not be great enough and the ball may not complete the diagonal of the court before touching the court floor.

1. A ceiling–front wall shot should hit the ceiling
   a. at the ceiling–front wall crotch.
   b. 2–3 feet from the ceiling–front wall crotch.
   c. after hitting the front wall.
   d. in the middle, halfway to the back wall.

2. The hardest court position to return a ball from is
   a. in the front court.
   b. in the middle of the service zone.
   c. just behind the short line.
   d. in a back corner close to both the back and side walls.

3. A ceiling–front wall shot can be hit
   a. from a ball below waist level.
   b. from a ball above your head.
   c. with both a forehand and backhand shot.
   d. all of the above.

4. If the front wall–ceiling shot is hit properly, it can be used to
   a. keep the ball in play.
   b. move your opponent to a back-court position.
   c. force a return that is not an offensive shot.
   d. all of the above.

5. A three-wall shot
   a. follows the path of a "V" across the court.
   b. is an offensive shot.
   c. is designed to rebound into the back court.
   d. all of the above.

6. The purpose of a defensive shot is to score a point.   T   F

7. Ideally, a defensive shot should rebound close to
   the front wall in the middle of the court.   T   F

8. The harder you hit a ceiling–front wall shot, the higher
   the height of the ball's bounce off the floor.   T   F

9. A ceiling–front wall shot can be hit from almost any court position.   T   F

10. To hit a lob shot correctly requires a strong, powerful stroke.   T   F

11. A ball hitting the floor before the back wall will have its
    rebound off the back wall slowed.   T   F

12. To hit a lob shot, return the ball low to the front wall.   T   F

13. A high-Z or three-wall shot is designed to move the
    opponent into a back corner.   T   F

14. An around-the-wall ball and a high Z both start with
    the ball rebounding off the front wall to a side wall.   T   F

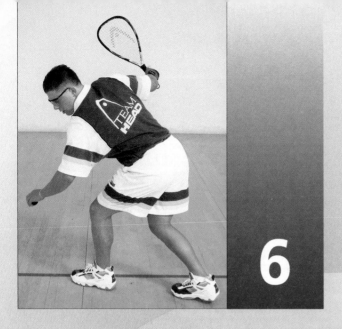

6

Serves in Racquetball

The serve is your best offensive weapon.

When serving, keep your opponent guessing.

Serving is the most important offensive weapon in the arsenal of a beginning player. The serve can either set up a winning shot or prevent the opponent from scoring on the return of serve. The effectiveness of the serve is due to the controlled way in which it can be hit. This is the only time when you can contact the ball in a position of your choosing. Thus, you can play to your strengths and/or your opponent's weaknesses if you can consistently serve your best shot.

There are only five basic serves. Each serve, however, can be changed to give a slightly different look by varying the power with which it is hit, its height of rebound off the front wall, and/or the angle of rebound into the back court. With these variations, the basic serves can become hundreds of different shots. The wise player mixes these variations to keep the opponent guessing as to where the next ball will be served. However, the serve chosen should be hit only after thought is given to an opponent's strengths and skills. Even a well-placed serve, if hit so an opponent can return it with a favorite shot, is nothing more than a nice setup. Similarly, a good

player never hits a weak serve merely for the sake of variety if it is not obvious an equally weak return will follow.

To make these serve variations effective, however, your serve must not become predictable, either from the position you take in the service zone or from the technique with which you strike the ball. Ideally, all serves should be hit from a similar position on the court, with a similar stroke. Usually the center of the service zone and a normal forehand stroke are used. In this way, it is difficult, if not impossible, for your opponent to anticipate the direction of your serve. This means that variation in your serve must be a result of the amount of wrist snap or the position of the racquet face at the moment of contact with the ball. Either factor will affect the angle of hit or the power of the stroke.

Since you as the server are the only one who knows where the serve will be hit, you also should anticipate the placement of the returned ball. So take the time before each serve to plan not only the best serve but also the most likely return and how best to play the ball. Ideally, if the serve is not an

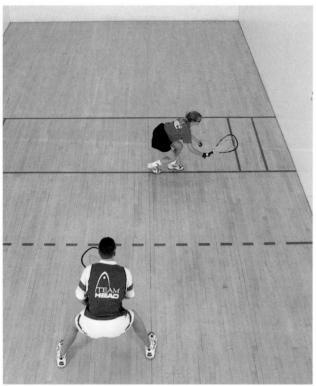

Figure 6.1 Serving position on the court.

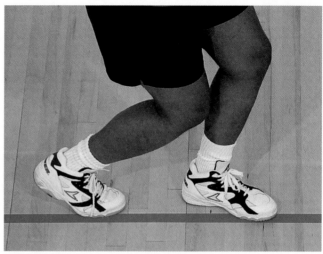

Figure 6.2 Foot placement to begin serve.

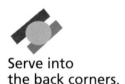

Serve into
the back corners.

outright winner, at least a poor return should result, setting you up for your best offensive stroke.

For an opponent whom you have never seen play, a good strategy is simply to serve to the backhand court with your best serve. If a player has a weakness, it is usually on the backhand side. This strategy should increase the odds of your winning the point with your serve.

The serve provides the server with the offensive advantage in the game. To serve without purpose or thought to your opponent's skill gives up this advantage and possibly the serve with it.

Legal Serves

For a serve to be a **legal serve**, the ball must be hit after it rebounds off the floor within the service zone. After contact with the racquet, the ball must strike the front wall before any other part of the court. However, the rebounding ball from the front wall may touch one side wall before falling to the floor

behind the short line. The ball may not touch the floor in front of the short line or on the short line (short), a second side wall (two-wall), the ceiling, or back wall (long) before the ball makes contact with the floor. A two-wall, short, long, or ceiling serve is an illegal serve (**fault**) and should not be played.

Most serves are hit with a forehand stroke. The server stands as far back as possible in the service zone with the hips pivoted to the side wall (see Figure 6.1). Both feet should be placed along the short line (see Figure 6.2). This provides as much service zone as possible in which to step forward when contacting the ball. Stepping out of the service zone during the serve is illegal (fault).

To begin the serve, the ball falls off the fingertips of the non-racquet hand and is dropped to the floor. The hand should be extended to the front wall so the ball is dropped as far forward as possible in the service zone (see Figure 6.3). If the ball is not dropped close to the service line (front part of the service zone), the server will move past the ball when stepping forward to hit it. Thus, contact with the ball will occur off the back foot, and much of the force of the stroke will be lost.

At the beginning of the serve, the racquet already has completed the

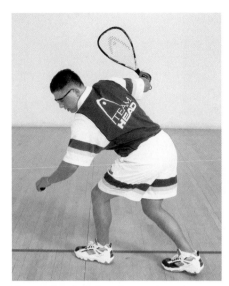

Figure 6.3 Ball drop for service.

"Handcuff" your opponent with a lob to the back corner.

FRONT

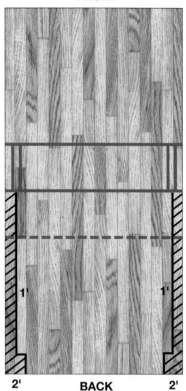

2'   **BACK**   2'

Figure 6.4 Optimal court areas for served ball to be directed.

backswing and is held perpendicular to the back wall. When the ball leaves the hand, the forward swing of the racquet begins. The angle of the racquet head and the height of the ball off the floor at contact are dependent upon the type of serve being hit. In any serve, however, it is essential to step into the stroke. Shifting the body's weight from the back of the service zone to the foot that steps toward the service line provides additional power.

The serve, as any other stroke, is completed with a follow-through, the final position of the racquet being dependent upon the type of serve used. It is important to always hit *through* the ball rather than merely punch at it. Although most serves are hit with a forehand stroke, on occasion a backhand or overhead stroke may be used.

The following five serves are designed to follow the rules of service as well as place the opponent in a poor court position from which to hit an

offensive return. As described with defensive strokes, this means hitting a ball into a back corner of the court. On all serves, it is important to keep the ball in the back corners and away from the midline of the court (see Figure 6.4). A return from the middle of the court provides too many opportunities for offensive shots and prevents the server from holding a center-court position. Thus, the following serves should be directed wide of the midline of the court and should rebound back to a center-court position only after bouncing twice on the floor and being ruled a dead ball. They are the lob, the drive, the Z, the overhead, and the garbage serves.

Lob

The **lob serve** is hit identically to the lob defensive shot, with the ball following the same path through the court (see Chapter 5). The serve may be hit crosscourt or down-the-line. As in the defensive lob, the ball must be hit high to the front wall, and the rebound should arc its way high over center court to die in a back-court corner. To do this, the forward swing of the stroke must involve the racquet face being held slightly open to the ceiling. The ball is contacted at waist level and hit high off the front wall. The stroke is finished with the racquet held high over the forward shoulder. As in the defensive lob, a lob serve requires finesse rather than power (see Figure 6.5).

To ensure that the ball will die in the back court, the lob serve can graze a side wall close to the back wall. This rebound will slow the movement of the ball. As a result, the serve must be directed accurately to a corner. Accuracy in placement is critical. If the ball does not "handcuff" your opponent in the back corner, this slow-moving ball will be an easy setup for an offensive return. If this is difficult for you to do, hit the serve to the opponent's backhand. This will provide for a margin of error in placement because it will force a weak-side return.

To increase the accuracy of the lob serve to the backhand side of the court, many players change their center-court serving position and move to that side

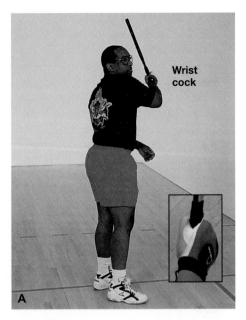

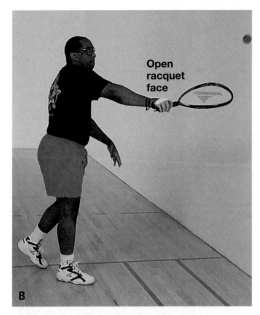

Wrist cock

Open racquet face

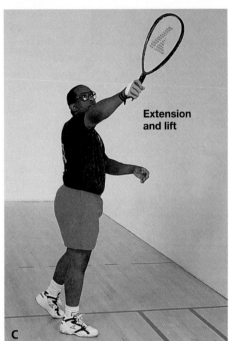

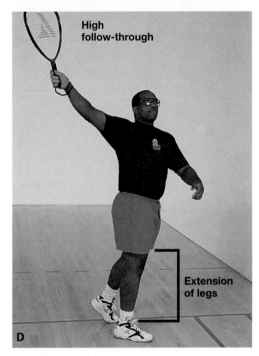

Extension and lift

High follow-through

Extension of legs

Figure 6.5 Backhand lob serve sequence.

of the service zone. In addition, they hit the ball with a backhand stroke, using an open racquet face as on the forehand side. Although there is little deception in this maneuver, the difficulty in returning a lob serve comes not in surprising the opponent as much as in placing the ball. This court position allows for better placement because the ball is not hit at an angle. Rather, the racquet is parallel to the front wall and the ball is hit straight.

The lob is a good serve to use to change the pace of the game and to slow down a fast-moving opponent who likes to return serves hard to the front wall. The lob can be varied by hitting the serve at a "half lob" position, i.e., one that is about shoulder height at the peak of its arc. Again, accuracy of placement is critical in the success of this serve.

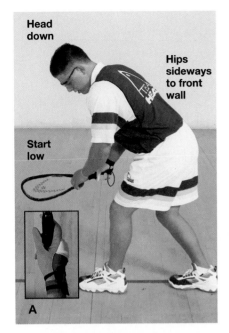

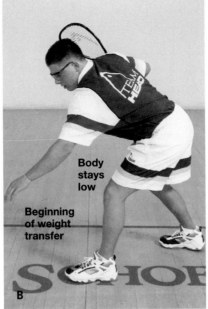

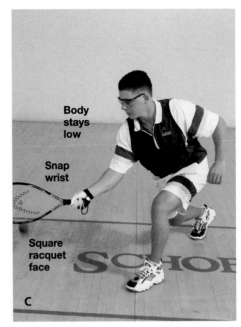

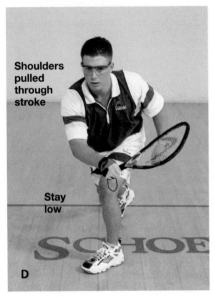

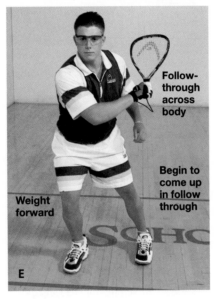

Figure 6.6
Drive serve sequence.

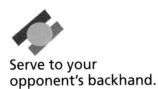

Serve to your
opponent's backhand.

Drive Serve

A **drive serve** is hit with a strong fore-hand stroke to ensure good speed on the ball. To maximize the power in the stroke, you must begin the serve with your hips sideways to the front wall and meet the ball by stepping toward it during the forward swing. The ball should be contacted close to the ground—somewhere between the bent knee and the ankle. The forward swing should be level to the ground and the ball met just inside the forward foot. The follow-through should be across the body and should pull the shoulders around to finish the stroke facing the front wall. This serve resembles the kill shot in technique (see Figure 6.6).

To be most effective, the drive serve must be hit low to the front wall to ensure a low ball rebounding into the back court. Keeping the ball low adds to the difficulty in the return.

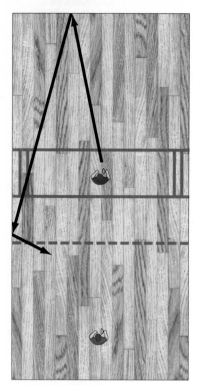

(a) behind the short line
Figure 6.7 Variations of drive serves.

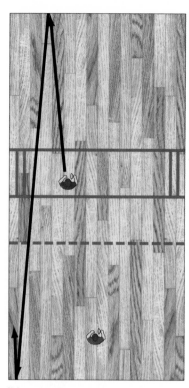

(b) to back corner

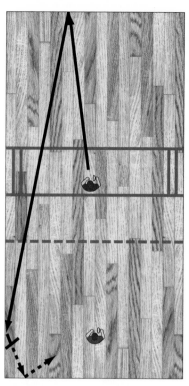

(c) off side wall

The drive serve is not directed to any one particular area of the court. As in other serves, however, the serve should not rebound close to the midline of the back court. As illustrated in Figure 6.7, the ball can (a) hit the side wall just past the short line (short corner drive serve), (b) go straight into the back corner of the court, or (c) hit the side wall several feet from the back wall and rebound around the back corner. Any of these serves will be effective as long as you vary the angle of rebound off the front wall from serve to serve and keep the ball low. To do this, the angle of the racquet face at ball contact must change with each hit. To prevent your opponent from anticipating the position of your serve, learn to hit a drive serve to the forehand and backhand sides of the court with equal skill. The backhand side is most effective in preventing offensive returns.

Z Serve

The **Z serve** can be divided into two distinct serves: a **high-Z serve** and a **low-Z serve**. The high-Z serve is similar to the defensive Z shot in its movement around the court. This serve hits high on the front wall close to the front wall–side wall crotch. The ball rebounds to the nearest side wall, then travels high across the diagonal of the court to the opposite back corner. For the serve to be legal, the ball must hit the floor before touching another wall (unlike the defensive Z shot) and rebounding again. Thus, the movement of the ball on the court resembles the letter "Z."

This Z serve is hit with the same technique as the defensive Z shot. The hips are turned to the side wall, the racquet face is open, and contact with the ball is made inside the forward foot. The stroke cannot be as strong as the defensive shot because the ball must touch the floor before striking the opposite side wall. Thus, like the lob serve, the high-Z serve requires proper placement and finesse, rather than power, to be effective.

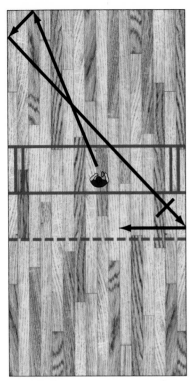

Figure 6.8 Low-Z serve hitting past short line.

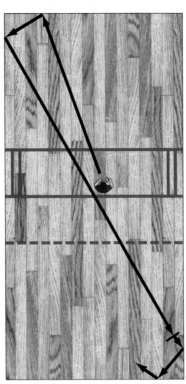

Figure 6.9 Low-Z serve directed to back corner of court.

At the opposite extreme, the low-Z serve requires power to make the shot work. The low-Z serve follows the same "Z" path around the court, but instead of traveling above shoulder height, the ball moves through the court close to the ground. Thus, this serve is hit low to the front wall, similar to the drive serve but with more strength because of the distance across the court the ball must travel (past the short line) before touching the floor.

The technique used to hit a low-Z serve is similar to that for a kill shot (see Chapter 4). The ball must be contacted inside the forward foot as the weight shifts forward. The racquet should have a level swing at contact with the ball, and the arm movement must be completed with a follow-through. Punching at the ball by stopping the racquet's motion after hitting the ball will limit the power of the swing. A good wrist snap is also essential in providing the power necessary to hit a low-Z ball.

The low Z may rebound to the floor anywhere along the side wall past the short line. If the ball is hit hard and close to the front wall–side wall crotch, the ball will rebound to the floor just behind the short line and hit the side wall (see Figure 6.8). The extreme spin on the ball, because of the power of the stroke, will cause the ball to rebound perpendicular to the side wall. An opponent positioned to hit a ball served deep into a back corner will be out of place to return this serve.

If the ball is hit several feet from the front wall–side wall crotch, the ball will be directed toward the back corner of the court (see Figure 6.9). The different angles that can be used to hit the low-Z serve depend on the angle of the racquet head when the ball is contacted. The variety of angles provides another means of preventing your opponent from knowing where to set up for the return of serve.

To be most successful, the low-Z serve requires a powerful and accurate stroke. If the ball is moving too slowly, the opponent may be tempted to hit the ball as it passes through the center-court position. For this reason, the low-Z serve is used primarily by experienced players and seldom by beginning players who have not mastered shifting their body weight and snapping the wrist to increase the power of the serve. Beginning players usually rely on the high-Z serve. Although this serve results in a slow-moving ball, it can be especially effective if hit to the backhand of a hard-hitting opponent because of its placement into a back corner.

Overhead Serve

The **overhead serve** is rarely used in competitive racquetball, but it is a legal serve. It is hit with a stroke similar to that used in an overhead kill (see Chapter 4), but the ball is not directed as low to the front wall as the kill shot is. The most difficult part of the stroke is starting the ball in play, since the ball must be hit only after rebounding off the floor. Therefore, to be contacted at a point over your head, the ball must hit the floor of the service zone with enough force so it rebounds above your head and outstretched arm. Thus, the ball must be thrown to the floor rather than dropped.

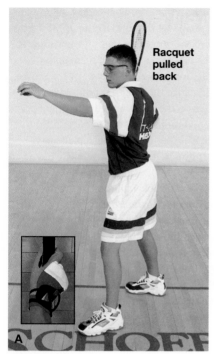
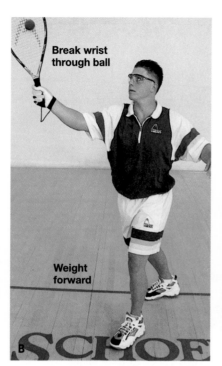
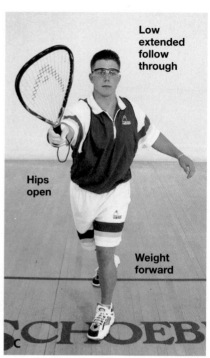

Racquet pulled back

Break wrist through ball

Low extended follow through

Hips open

Weight forward

Weight forward

Figure 6.10 Overhead serve sequence.

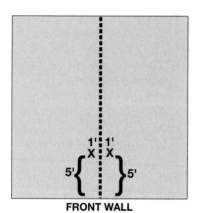

FRONT WALL

Figure 6.11 Target area on front wall for overhead serve.

Never serve down the middle of the court.

Because this throw must be done with your non-racquet (non-dominant) hand, the throw is difficult to make. If the ball is not thrown straight down, it will rebound out of the service area rather than overhead and cannot be hit. If the ball is not thrown with enough force, it will not bounce high enough for a proper overhead stroke.

Therefore, if you anticipate using an overhead serve in a game, you should practice the throw until its placement is consistent. If the throw is done correctly, the overhead stroke should contact the ball just inside the forward foot with the racquet held in an extended arm.

To hit the ball with the most control, the server should use a Western grip. The backswing and forward swing of the stroke resembles a circle, much like a tennis serve. The ball should be contacted at a point overhead after you have stepped onto your forward foot and shifted your body weight forward onto the ball of this foot. Until the point of impact, the racquet face should trail the wrist. Upon contact with the ball, the wrist and racquet should be snapped forward to direct the ball toward the bottom third of the front wall. This

snapping not only will direct the ball downward but also will increase the force of the stroke. The overhead serve is completed with a follow-through that brings the racquet downward (see Figure 6.10).

The ball should hit the front wall 5 to 6 feet off the floor. This will ensure a low rebound into the back court. If the serve is hit lower, the ball will hit the floor in front of the short line and be called a fault. To rebound into a back corner, the ball must contact the front wall at least 1 foot on either side of the center when you are serving from the middle of the service zone (see Figure 6.11). The overhead serve offers no unique advantage except a different look. Some beginning players like to hit an overhead serve because of its similarity to a tennis serve, with which they are familiar and can hit with power. However, the most difficult serves to return are not necessarily the most powerful but, rather, those that are placed most accurately and rebound low into a back-corner position.

Because the ball is hit down to the front wall with an overhead serve, the ball often will rebound off the floor with a high bounce (see Figure 6.12). Thus,

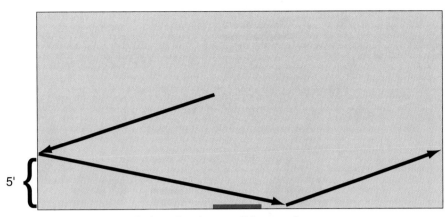

5'

Figure 6.12 Rebound of overhead serve off front wall.

the ball may not be close to the floor in the back court. Keeping the ball low to the floor on the serve, as done with the drive or low Z, is more effective. This is why experienced players prefer these serves.

Garbage Serve

A **garbage serve** is hit with a forehand stroke. This serve looks much like a drive serve. The forward swing is level with the floor, and the ball is contacted inside the front foot. The force of the hit is dependent upon the speed of the swing and the snap of the wrist when the ball is contacted. The ball should not be hit as hard as it is in a drive serve, or as softly as a lob. Yet, the follow-through should draw the racquet across the body to hit "through the ball." Although the ball should rebound wide of the midline of the court, it is not hit low to the floor or high to the ceiling. Rather, the ball rebounds into the back court at a height between the opponent's waist and shoulder level off the floor. To hit the ball to this height, the server must contact the ball at a point higher off the floor than for a drive serve or with the racquet face slightly open. In general, the movement of the ball on the court gives the impression that the ball has been mis-hit.

This serve may or may not be hit with enough angle to rebound off a side wall before entering the back court. If it is, the ball should just brush the side wall so the ball does not rebound back into play. In this respect, a garbage serve is similar to a half lob.

If the serve is directed straight into the back corner, the ball must not be hit hard enough to rebound strongly off the back wall after hitting the floor. A strong rebound at this point will negate the value of the garbage serve. The strategy behind this serve is to force a ceiling return or prevent your opponent from hitting a kill shot or other offensive return. This strategy is especially effective with an opponent who can hit offensive shots consistently off your best serve, placing you immediately on the defensive. Using a garbage serve should at least get you past the serve and onto other opportunities to win the point.

Points to Remember

→ Unless a serve requires a different court position, serve from the center of the service zone with a forehand stroke so you don't signal the type of serve you will hit.

→ Never serve the ball down the midline of the court, where an offensive return is easy to hit.

→ In addition to hitting the serve wide of the middle of the court, hit the ball low unless a garbage serve, lob, or high Z is desired.

→ Serve to the backhand side of the court if you don't know your opponent.

→ Practice serving to the righthand side of the court in case you play a left-handed player (this will be the backhand side) and to provide variation in your serve.

→ Practice hitting your serves to rebound at different angles off the front wall, using varying heights off the floor and changing the power in your stroke.

→ The closer to the center of the front wall the ball is hit, the farther back in the court the ball will strike a side wall. The closer to a front wall corner the ball strikes, the closer to the front wall the ball will hit the side wall.

→ Use a lob or high-Z serve to change the pace of the game or to force a ceiling ball return.

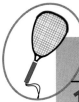

Common Errors and How to Correct Them

1. **My lob serve hits the ceiling or the back wall.**

You are hitting the ball too hard or with too much angle toward the ceiling. Hit the ball softer and with less angle so the ball will hit lower on the front wall.

2. **My drive serve rebounds off the back wall into the center court.**

Bend your knees, bringing your body closer to the floor so you can drop your racquet lower to the floor. This will allow you to contact the ball when it is closer to the floor. Hitting a lower ball into the back court will lessen the chance of a rebound off the back wall. In addition, angling the ball to hit a side wall before it touches the back court floor should deaden the movement of the ball into the back court and prevent a hard rebound from the back wall.

3. **My Z serve hits two side walls before it hits the floor.**

Hit the ball farther from the front corner and closer to the center of the front wall so the ball will rebound to a point farther into the back court. Another correction would be to hit the ball with less stroking power while keeping the same forward swing to maintain the height of the ball's contact with the front wall.

4. **My drive serve pops off the front wall and rebounds high into the back court.**

You probably are standing up as you make contact with the ball during the serve. If you do not maintain a low position to the floor throughout the forward swing, the ball will be lifted along with your body and rebound up off the front wall. Make sure that you have followed through your serving motion before you come to a ready position to prepare for the return of serve.

5. **My garbage serve hits straight into the back wall.**

You are hitting the serve too hard. Take some power off your stroke, and angle the racquet head slightly toward the ceiling upon contact with the ball.

6. **My serves go straight down the center of the court.**

You are not hitting the ball with enough angle (toward a front wall corner). This can be corrected in one of two ways: (1) If you want to hit the ball to the side wall behind you, throw the ball out in front of you toward your backhand side. If you want to hit the ball toward the side wall you are facing, throw the ball slightly behind the front foot and toward your forehand side. (2) If you want to serve to the side wall behind, you always throw the ball in the same place relative to your body, but concentrate on breaking your wrist upon contact with the ball. If you want to hit toward the side wall you are facing, open up your wrist (laid-back position). This technique is the best because it will disguise your service direction until contact is made.

7. **My overhead serve always hits the floor in front of the short line.**

You are hitting the ball too low to the front wall. Check to see if you are hitting the ball just inside your forward foot and if your racquet head is angled in the direction in which you want the ball to go. If so, you must aim at a higher point off the floor for the ball to contact the front wall. To do this, don't snap your wrist as much when contacting the ball, or hit the ball when it is at a higher point on its rebound, or both.

?????

Self Testing Questions

Answers to Self Testing Questions are located on page 131.

1 A service fault is called

    a. when the ball strikes the front wall, then a side wall.
    b. when the ball hits the back-wall crotch.
    c. when the ball touches the ceiling after the front wall.
    d. when the ball is hit with an overhead stroke.

2. A lob serve can be used to

    a. change the pace of the game.
    b. overpower your opponent.
    c. slow down a hard-hitting opponent.
    d. "handcuff" an opponent against a side wall.

3. All serves should avoid

    a. hitting the back wall before the floor.
    b. rebounding into the middle of the court.
    c. hitting the floor before the ball passes the short line.
    d. all of the above.

4. Ideally, all serves should be hit from a similar position in the service zone with a similar stroke to prevent your opponent from predicting the placement of your serve.   T   F

5. Beginning players usually hit their weakest returns from the backhand side.   T   F

6. A lob serve is most effective if hit close to a side wall.   T   F

7. To be most effective, a drive serve should be hit high off the front wall.   T   F

8. In order to keep your opponent guessing where your serve will go, you can vary the angle of the rebound off the front wall, the rebound height off the front wall, and how hard the ball is hit.   T   F

9. A low-Z serve is used primarily by beginning players as one of their first serves.   T   F

10. The overhead serve offers no unique advantage over any other serve.   T   F

11. Serving provides you with your best opportunity to control the game.   T   F

12. For a serve to be legal, it must hit the floor before hitting the front wall.   T   F

13. A serve that doesn't rebound when you want it to is referred to as a "garbage" serve.   T   F

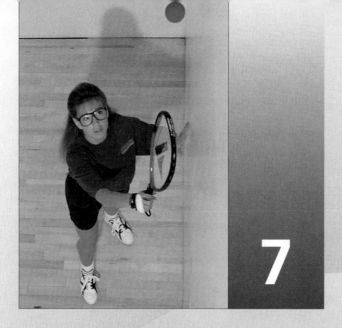

7

Special Strokes and Shots

A ball hit into the back wall: run forward.

Offensive and defensive strokes comprise the primary skills involved in the game of racquetball, but additional skills are needed to play the game to your advantage. These skills include hitting off the back wall, hitting into the back wall, corner-shot returns, drop shots, and the volley.

The Back Wall

Up to now, this book has ignored the part of racquetball that makes it an interesting and challenging game—use of the **back wall**. Beginning players often learn to play racquetball by avoiding the back wall completely. As a result, they are not really playing four-wall racquetball. This type of play puts these players at a disadvantage when facing opponents who use the whole court. Without using the back wall as a playable surface, two problems arise: (1) any ball that gets past your position in the court is out of play with no chance for you to retrieve it, and (2) to prevent balls from getting past them, players use unorthodox strokes with unpredictable results to return the ball. Thus, when not using the back wall, players often

must resort to merely hitting the ball to keep it in play rather than directing it. We refer to this strategy as "Battleball."

When playing Battleball, the player maintains a center-court position and hits every ball within reach as hard as possible back to the middle of the front wall. The strategy is that if the ball is hit hard to the front wall, it may rebound past the opponent and score a point. Of course, this tactic may work against another Battleball player, but the experienced opponent will use the back wall skillfully to keep the ball in play. Only until you feel confident enough to use the back wall will you be able to play more than Battleball on the racquetball court.

Patience

The key to using the back wall effectively is *patience*—the patience to let a ball intentionally go past you. Before you can play with patience, you must develop confidence in your ability to play balls on the rebound off the back wall. Part of this confidence comes from many hours of court practice and another part from understanding why the back wall is helpful.

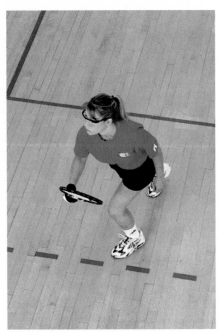

Figure 7.1 Moving for a back wall return.

"Ride with the ball" off the back wall.

Back Wall Advantage

Use of the back wall is important because it provides several advantages during the game. First, a ball that goes past you into the back court can still be hit as it rebounds off the back wall.

Second, by waiting for balls to rebound off the back wall, you can move into a better position for hitting a forehand or backhand stroke—the setup for the return. If the ball is hit before the back wall rebound, often it is above or below the ideal hitting area. It is impossible to practice hitting balls at all positions relative to your body. Thus, always adjusting your court position so the ball is at the same place relative to your forehand or backhand stroke will ensure a consistent hit. This means you will be in control of the ball's movement around the court and, consequently, your opponent's court position as well. Finally, waiting for the rebound affords you more time to see where your opponent is waiting in the court and to plan the most effective offensive return. Thus, use of the back wall adds to your ability to control movement of the ball and your opponent's court position and to potentially gain an offensive advantage.

Getting in Position

To position yourself to hit a good return off the back wall, you must never lose eye contact with the ball or turn your back to the front wall (see Figure 7.1). The most critical mistake that players make when returning balls off the back wall is turning to face the back wall when stroking the ball. As a result, a normal forehand or backhand stroke cannot be used because the ball would be hit into the side wall. Thus, out of desperation, the player facing the back wall resorts to flipping the ball over the shoulder, hitting a blind shot toward the front. This shot does not allow you to control and direct the movement of the ball—only to keep it in play. The only way to use the back wall successfully is to pivot your hips for a forehand or backhand return and adjust your position relative to the ball's rebound by cross-stepping up or back.

The critical decision to be made when returning a ball from the back wall is whether to use a forehand or a backhand shot. This decision must be made quickly, and the pivot to the appropriate side should follow immediately. It is easy to judge the side from which most balls should be hit. Balls that follow the diagonal of the court, however, are more difficult to play. Usually these balls begin in the front court and end in the back court at the opposite corner. Therefore, a ball that begins on your left side becomes a hit from the right side, and you must pivot to the opposite corner from where the ball rebounds in the front court. Practicing for these balls on the court is the best way to learn how to position yourself.

To hit any ball off the back wall properly, a player never can afford to stop watching the ball as it rebounds off the front wall for the back wall hit. Follow the ball from your pivot position, moving only your eyes to keep the ball in sight.

Once the pivot to the appropriate side has been made, proper positioning for the rebound will allow you to either make or miss the shot. It is hard to learn how to adjust your position for the ball without going into the court and practicing, but a few general guidelines may be helpful in getting you started.

If the ball has touched the floor before it hits the back wall, you must hit it before it touches the floor again, directly off the rebound. Because it has touched the floor, the ball's bounce is deadened and will not rebound far off the back wall (see Figure 7.2). Thus, you

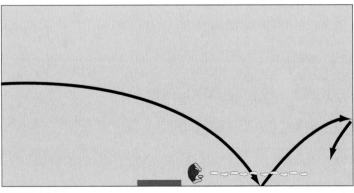

Figure 7.2 Move to the back court to return a ball rebounding off back wall after hitting court floor.

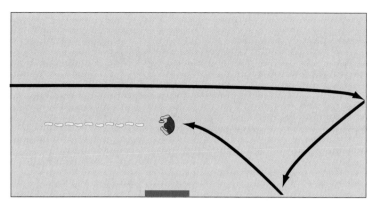

Figure 7.3 Move to center court to return ball rebounding off back wall.

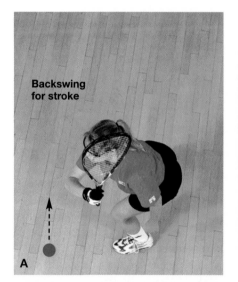

Backswing for stroke

A

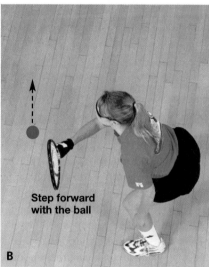

Step forward with the ball

B

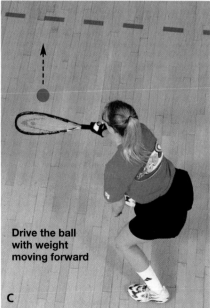

Drive the ball with weight moving forward

C

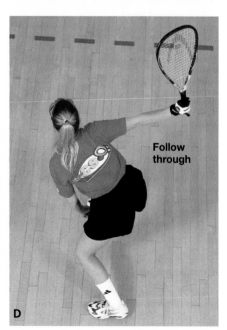

Follow through

D

Figure 7.4 Backhand return off back wall.

will need to move close to the back wall to hit the ball. If the ball hits the back wall without touching the floor, you should wait for the ball to hit the floor before making contact with it. But be prepared to move forward in the court, because the ball will rebound sharply off the wall and run toward the front-court area (see Figure 7.3). In either case, you need to position yourself so that at the point of contact, the ball will be hit inside the forward foot with the proper forehand or backhand stroking motion (see Figure 7.4).

A more difficult shot to return is the back-wall rebound of a lob or ceiling shot that just grazes the back wall, dies, and falls to the floor. With either shot, the ball has touched the floor already. Therefore, the ball must be hit immediately after contact with the back wall. The only way to hit this type of rebound successfully is with a sharp wrist snap on the racquet. Station the racquet between the path of the ball and the wall (see Figure 7.5). As the ball passes the face of the racquet, flip the racquet forward with a sharp wrist motion. The best return on this ball is a defensive shot directed toward the top of the front wall. This way, if the shot is weak, the ball still will make contact somewhere on the front wall surface. In addition, a defensive return will give you time to reposition yourself on the court.

If, during a game, you are not able to return the ball off the back wall, you may have to hit the ball as it is falling toward you, before it strikes the back wall. In this case, the best shot to use is an overhead ceiling shot (see Chapter 5). With this return, you will keep the ball in play and have an opportunity to win the rally later.

Never jump to hit these balls. All balls eventually will fall to within arm's reach. If the ball hits so high off the back wall that it can't be hit with an outstretched arm, wait for the rebound. Jumping only adds another factor to control when trying to hit the ball perfectly. Jumping for the ball is a sign of impatience.

Points to Remember

→ Watch the ball at all times.
  → To hit a ball off the back wall, pivot 90° to the side from which the shot is to be taken, and cross-step forward or backward to a court position where the ball will rebound.
  → If the ball touches the floor before the back wall, the rebound will drop close to the back wall.
  → If the ball hits the back wall before touching the floor, the ball will rebound into a mid- to center-court position.
→ Return balls that rebound strongly off the back wall with a defensive or an offensive shot using either a backhand or a forehand stroke.
→ Return a ball that grazes the back wall by emphasizing the wrist snap and placing the racquet along the wall, hitting a defensive return as the ball falls past the face of the racquet.

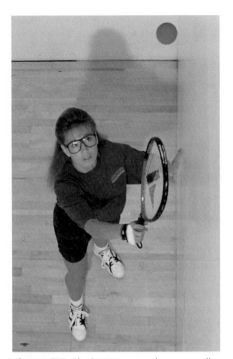

Figure 7.5 Placing racquet close to wall to hit ball.

Never jump to hit the ball.

Hitting into the Back Wall

Rather than using the back wall properly, a temptation for a beginning player is to hit the ball into the back wall with the hope that it will rebound the length of the court to the front wall. This type of hit is more likely to happen if the player turns completely around to face the back wall when playing the rebound. For some players, hitting into the back wall becomes a favorite shot. Unfortunately, the more you rely on this shot, the weaker your game will be.

First, it is impossible to hit an offensive shot off an into-the-back-wall hit. Second, even defensive shots are unreliable from this return because you are facing away from the front wall, making it almost impossible to aim the ball. Finally, with the distance the ball must travel (more than the full length of the court), the ball becomes a slow-moving, easy target for your opponent to return. Hitting the ball into the back wall, then, should be used only as a last resort when there is no other way to keep the ball in play.

The only two occasions in which this situation is likely to occur (short of your moving lazily to a good court position) are (1) off a passing shot that

beats you into the back court, and (2) a ball that falls so close to the back wall from a ceiling, lob, or served ball that you cannot place your racquet between it and the wall to stroke it forward.

If a back-wall return must be used, be sure to contact the ball with an upward scooping motion to angle the rebound above your head and high toward the front wall. The ball must be hit hard.

Never hit the ball into the back wall from a mid- or center-court position. Not only is this bad strategy, but your opponent may be in the back court and, consequently, in the path of the ball. Standing 10–15 feet away from a hit ball gives your opponent little time to duck. Many serious injuries have resulted from this type of play.

The player who wants to win at racquetball cannot afford to rely on such an ineffective and dangerous shot. To avoid placing yourself in the position of hitting the ball into the back wall: (1) never turn 180° to face the back wall to return a ball, and (2) move quickly to meet the ball in the court rather than be caught out of position with no other shot available.

A ball that bounces on the floor: go back.

Use a wrist snap with a corner ball.

Corner Shots

Another important return to learn is hitting a ball that rebounds to a back corner. For most players, the **corner shot** return is the most difficult play in the game. To contact a corner ball, you must contend with the back and side walls simultaneously. Without any room to stroke the ball, an effective offensive shot is eliminated, and you can hope only for a good defensive return.

To play a corner shot, it is important to pivot immediately toward the corner in which the ball will rebound while keeping the ball in view. The success of this return is dependent upon your ability to position yourself properly in relation to the ball's movement. Anticipate the ball's rebound, and maintain a court position behind the forward bounce. From this position you still can step into the ball to make contact. If the ball does not rebound with enough force to allow you to hit the ball with a forward swing, the power in the hit must come primarily from the wrist snap (see Figure 7.6).

The last option to keep the ball in play is to hit the ball into the back wall with enough strength to have it rebound to the front wall. This strategy has been discussed previously.

The key to a successful corner shot return is having the patience to wait for the ball to rebound off the back wall. Most beginners do not have the patience to wait, and they swing wildly as the ball comes within reach. Another mistake commonly made is using a wide, sweeping swing with an extended arm, using the shoulder to supply the force behind the stroke. Not only is this big arm swing dangerous, but there is no room for this type of tennis stroke in the corner of the court.

Contact with a ball in the corner that has little rebound off the back wall should be made with an open racquet face. This will direct the ball toward the ceiling and give you more margin for error. If the ball rebounds away from the back wall, any forehand or backhand return can be used. Most players, however, choose a defensive return because of their back-court position. Therefore, the return of a corner ball should be considered successful if a good defensive shot is hit.

Points to Remember

→ Hit into the back wall rarely. This is a desperation shot and provides little advantage to the player except to keep the ball in play.

→ Never hit into the back wall from a center- or mid-court position.

→ When returning the ball to the back wall, use a scooping stroke to lift the ball over your head and past your face.

→ Hit the ball hard, as it must travel more than the length of the court.

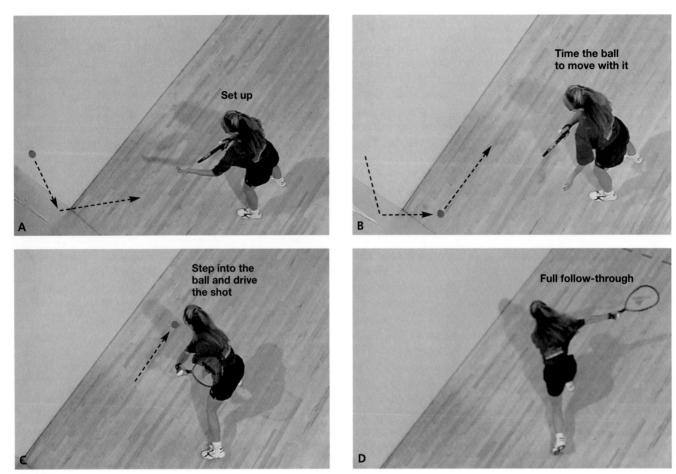

Figure 7.6 Hitting out of corner sequence.

Points to Remember

→ For all corner shots, position yourself behind the rebound so you can step into the ball to return it.
→ Avoid using a big arm swing, especially if the ball is rebounding tightly into the corner; instead, rely on a wrist snap.
→ If the ball does not rebound strongly out of the corner, hit a defensive ceiling shot rather than try for an offensive return.
→ Return a ball that rebounds hard off the corner with any type of shot.

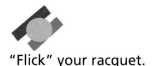

"Flick" your racquet.

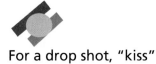

For a drop shot, "kiss" the ball.

Drop Shot

The **drop shot** is an offensive shot that requires placement, timing, and deception. Therefore, it is not considered a shot for novice players. The drop shot can be hit with either a forehand or a backhand stroke. Most players find this shot most successful if using it from a front-court position. This is true especially when their opponent is caught in the back court.

Often the player is not positioned in the front court for the shot but has to move there from a center-court position with the intent of hitting a drop shot. Therefore, the best ball from which to hit a drop shot is one that rebounds off the back wall and runs to the front court. Consequently, the player must follow the ball into the front court to return it.

The deception in a drop shot is that it looks like any other hard-hit stroke. The opponent expects the ball to rebound quickly off the front wall. At the point of contact, however, the forward swing is slowed and the face of the racquet is opened. The ball is "kissed" with just enough force to return it to the front. The deadened hit results in a rebound that drops immediately to the floor. If the opponent is in the back court or even center court, a well-executed drop shot will not be returned.

To ensure success of the drop shot, try to hit the ball to a front corner. If the ball makes contact with both the front wall and a side wall, its movement naturally will be deadened. Thus, a ball hit with too much force will still slow and drop quickly to the floor.

If your opponent follows you to the front court in anticipation of a drop shot, you can still win the point by hitting away at the ball. A hard, low rebound off the front wall will catch your opponent moving in the wrong direction. Using a drop shot or hitting the ball with a strong stroke is determined by your opponent's court position.

Points to Remember

→ For the most success, hit a drop shot from a front-court position.

→ Hit the ball into the corner to ensure that the ball will die quickly after the return.

→ Set up your drop shot as if it is going to be a hard-hit return, but upon contact with the ball, slow the forward swing and hold the racquet face in an open position.

Volley

By definition, a **volley** is a shot in which the ball is hit after it rebounds from the front wall and before it touches the floor. Consequently, any shot can be hit as a volley with either a forehand or a backhand stroke. Ideally, you must still pivot when volleying the ball, to ensure a proper stroke on the return. A volleyed ball, however, is often a mis-hit because the player has not set up properly for a defensive or offensive shot. Thus, the ball is hit with an unorthodox stroke and loses its effectiveness. This problem occurs because of the ball's quick rebound off the front wall, which allows little time to set up properly for the return. Therefore, hitting a good volley is not as dependent upon moving to the ball as it is upon the ball rebounding to the appropriate court position to allow you time to hit it. Thus, every ball is not a good prospect for a volley return.

Unfortunately, beginning players often volley a return to avoid (1) moving to a correct position to hit a ball, or (2) returning balls that would rebound off the back wall. Experienced players volley a return with one of three strategies in mind: (1) to change the pace of the game by speeding up the return to the front wall; (2) to avoid having the ball rebound into a court position (corner) that would make a strong return impossible; or (3) to force an opponent to hit a return before he/she can set up properly for the ball.

The third strategy is executed most effectively if the ball is returned directly to the opponent. As a result of this return, the opponent typically is handcuffed. The ball rebounds so quickly to the player's position that there is no time to get the racquet head moving to hit the ball. Therefore, the experienced player chooses to hit a volley for a strategic reason rather than because the ball merely rebounds within reach.

Beginning players hitting a volley with an overhead stroke should direct the ball either to the ceiling for a defensive shot or directly to the front wall in an attempt to pass the opponent. More experienced players may return an overhead kill.

A volleyed ball hit from a position low off the floor provides an opportunity to hit a kill shot return. Even beginning players may attempt this offensive volley with a low rebounding ball, especially if they are holding a center- or mid-court position.

Use a volley to "handcuff" your opponent.

Hit a volley for a reason, not to avoid moving on the court.

Points to Remember

→ Do not volley to avoid using the back wall but, rather, to change the pace of the game, catch your opponent out of position, or avoid a more difficult shot.
→ Before volleying a ball, position yourself correctly for a backhand, forehand, or overhead shot.

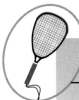

Common Errors and How to Correct Them

1. **When I try to return a ball from a back corner, my racquet always hits a side wall.**

You are using a large arm swing to hit the ball rather than relying on the wrist snap. Place the racquet along the anticipated path of the ball, and contact the ball when it moves past the racquet face, using a sharp wrist snap.

2. **When I hit a rebound off the back wall, my return always hits a side wall.**

Check to see if you are turning your hips to face the back wall rather than making only a pivot toward the side wall. This body position will cause you to hit the ball into a side wall rather than forward.

When hitting the ball, the racquet face also may be directed at a side wall if you are contacting the ball either off your back foot or too far in front of your forward foot. Try repositioning yourself when hitting a back-wall shot so contact with the ball is made in proper position relative to your body for the stroke you are using.

3. **My drop shots rebound off the front wall and into the court for an easy return by my opponent.**

You are hitting your drop shot with too much force. Slow your forward swing more or try hitting the ball lower to the front wall and into a corner. With a low corner ball, even a hard-hit drop shot should rebound quickly to the floor and out of your opponent's reach.

4. **When I try to volley a return, I always hit the side wall first.**

You either are keeping your hips parallel to the front wall when stroking the ball across your body to a side wall, or you are reacting too slowly to the ball. When reacting too slowly, the ball will be hit too far behind you. In this position, the racquet face has not been snapped in to the proper angle to hit the ball back to the front wall and the ball is returned at an angle.

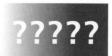

Self Testing Questions

Answers to Self Testing Questions are located on page 131.

1. Using the back wall allows you to
    a. return balls that go past you in the court.
    b. move to a better position to return a ball.
    c. note your opponent's position and hit where he/she is not.
    d. all of the above.

2. To be effective, the drop shot requires
    a. timing and deception.
    b. power of stroke.
    c. a forehand stroke.
    d. all of the above.

3. Experienced players will hit a volley return to
    a. change the pace of the game.
    b. prevent the ball from rebounding into the corner.
    c. force the opponent to hit a return before he/she is prepared.
    d. all of the above.

4. A good player should avoid hitting the ball directly into the back wall unless absolutely necessary.   T   F

5. A ball can best be hit if it is struck at the highest point off the floor, even if you have to jump to hit it.   T   F

6. Balls that rebound into the corner of the court should be hit with a full arm swing because you must generate a lot of force to hit them back to the front wall.   T   F

7. The drop shot is an offensive shot.   T   F

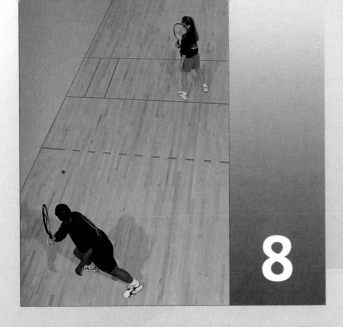

8

Putting the Strokes Together: Non-Thinking Strategy

As a beginning player on the court, your strategy is limited by your skill level. As you become more proficient with a variety of shots and feel confident enough to use them in a game situation, your strategy will change accordingly. With limited playing skills, however, success on the court is obtained most easily using a defensive strategy. This means that your objective during each rally is to keep the ball in play with defensive shots while maintaining a good court position. Points are won with this strategy, not because you make an outstanding offensive shot but, instead, because your opponent makes errors in his/her return.

At the beginning level, unforced errors account for more than half of the points scored. Therefore, if you can keep the ball in play with defensive shots, the odds are on your side that your opponent will lose the rally. This may not be as satisfying as hitting a winning shot, but it is more productive in the end. This is called the **non-thinking strategy** because few decisions are made during play. The only decision you must make is *which* defensive shot to hit.

Why are defensive shots a good choice for a beginning player? Simply because these shots are easiest to learn

and consistently hit correctly. Defensive shots can be hit hard or soft from anywhere on the court, and there is more room for error in their placement while still being strategically effective. To play a defensive game successfully, several points should be remembered.

Concentrate and Watch the Ball

To follow any strategy when playing racquetball, you must *concentrate* on the game and *watch the ball* (see Figure 8.1). Leave any mental distractions outside the court to improve your concentration on the game, for the players' safety and the fun of the game. A player who is distracted by other thoughts may end up at the painful end of a well-placed stroke, or at the very least missing easy-to-hit shots.

Part of concentrating on the game requires that you watch the ball at all times (see Figure 8.2). This is true regardless of whether or not it is your turn to hit the ball. The movement of the ball is so fast around the court, with the potential to change directions quickly, that losing eye contact with the ball usually results in an inability to properly

83

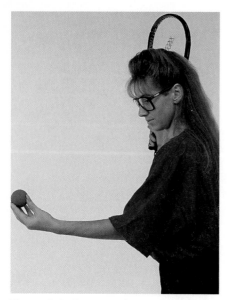

Figure 8.1 Concentrating and watching the ball.

Serve to a corner.

set up for the stroke in time. Therefore, your return may result in loss of a point simply because of your poor court position.

Serve Your Best

Even though you are following a defensive strategy, you can and should use your serve to its offensive advantage. This means *serve your best*. "Best" can be defined in two ways: (1) the serve you hit well with predictable results, or (2) the serve that may not be hit skillfully but attacks the opponent's weakness in service return.

How would you choose between these two options? Usually the choice is automatic. If a particular type of serve (such as lob to the backhand side) always gains a point for you through a faulty return, use it. If your opponent has no consistent weakness with one type of serve, use your most skilled serve—one that always is placed properly and hit with authority.

Unfortunately, when playing a new opponent, it will take time and possibly some lost serves before you can discover a player's weakness or which serve is working best for you that day. In this case, a good strategy is to serve to

the opponent's backhand. For most beginning players, the backhand suffers from a lack of practice because forehand strokes are hit with more success. Therefore, backhand strokes are not as skillfully controlled.

In addition to hitting toward the backhand side, the effectiveness of any serve can be increased if the ball is hit so the rebound lands close to a side wall in a back corner (see Figure 8.3). This court position makes the serve more difficult to return with an offensive stroke. Another benefit of this serve placement is that your opponent must move from the middle of the court to return the ball. Consequently, this court position is open for you to occupy.

If you still are confused as to how to serve the ball, use your own experience as a guide. The serve that is most difficult for you to return will be the most difficult for your opponent as well, assuming that both of you are at similar skill levels. Your service strategy does not suggest that a serve is successful only if it is an **ace**. Rather, the serve is useful if a weak return (a ball that is neither an offensive nor a good defensive shot) follows. This type of return sets you up for an easy offensive shot to the front wall and a point.

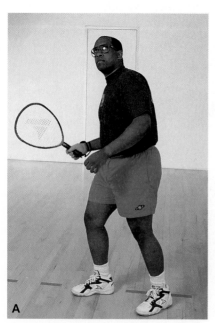
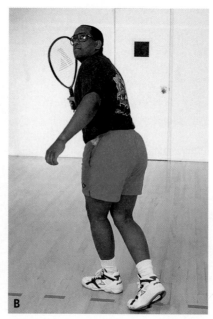
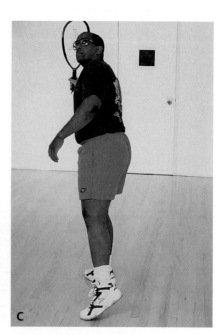

A   B   C

Figure 8.2 Moving and watching the ball.

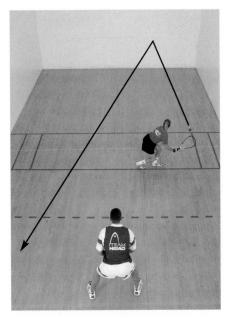

Figure 8.3 Serving to back corner.

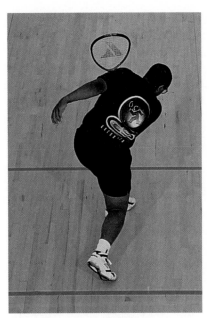

Figure 8.4 Service position in service zone.

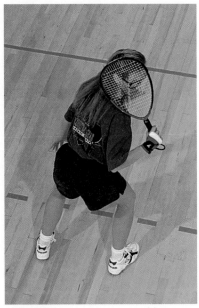

Figure 8.5 Center-court position, safely watching the ball.

Keep a Center-Court Position

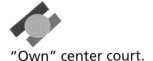

"Own" center court.

In a game involving beginning players, balls often pass through the center court after rebounding off the front wall. This is because the novice player returns most balls to the center of the front wall. Therefore, standing 1 to 3 feet behind the short line and an equal distance from either side wall will give you the best position to reach most balls. A **center-court position** is suggested not only because more balls travel through this area than any other part of the court, but because from here the player can reach balls that rebound short or long or run along either wall.

How do you gain and maintain this strategic center-court position? If you are serving, the problem is solved easily. When playing singles, the server usually serves from a position close to the center of the service zone (see Figure 8.4). This position is taken for two reasons. First, if all serves are hit from the same place in the service zone, there is little chance of the server's court position giving away the type of serve that is going to be hit. Second, this position allows easy access to the strategic playing position in center court.

As soon as the server is allowed to leave the service zone, this player should back up into the center court. Because of the server's proximity to center court, a few quick steps will do the job. Unfortunately, beginning players often choose to turn, face the back wall (and the receiver who is hitting the ball), and move to a center-court position while watching the serve. Not only is this dangerous because it exposes the server to a direct "in-the-face" return off the receiver's racquet, but a quick return of serve also may find the server's back to the front wall as the ball rebounds. Backing up to center court while using peripheral vision to follow the ball (see Figure 8.5) is the safest and the most effective tactic.

Maintaining this court position after the serve is merely a matter of keeping your opponent out of it. To do this, place your shots consistently so the rebound off the front wall is wide of the middle of the court and deep into a back-court position. A ceiling, lob, or high-Z ball are all effective in placing the ball deep into a back-court corner. To return these shots, your opponent

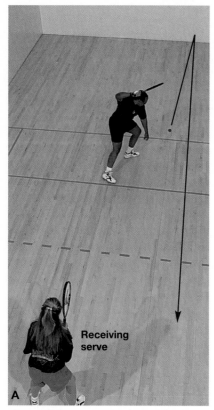

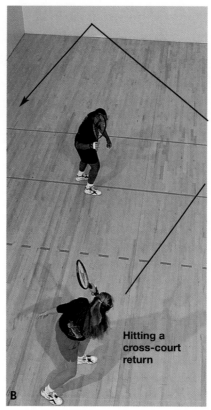

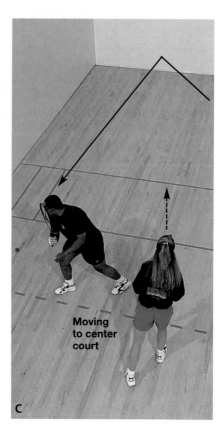

A — Receiving serve

B — Hitting a cross-court return

C — Moving to center court

Figure 8.6 Moving the server out of a center-court position.

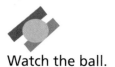

Watch the ball.

must follow the ball to the back court, leaving the center-court position open for you to occupy. As long as your returns are hit in this manner, the center court always will be open.

One precaution that beginners must be aware of is to avoid hitting the ball hard enough to allow it to rebound off the back wall and into the center court. Since the player hitting the ball cannot be impeded by the opponent, a rebound of this type would force you to move out of a center-court position.

Similarly, if you are receiving the serve, hitting a defensive stroke (such as the ceiling, lob, or high Z) along a side wall into a back corner or even a cross-court return will open the center court as the server chases your return (see Figure 8.6). Therefore, you should be

ready to move to the center-court position once your opponent has vacated this area. The usual movement on a racquetball court consists of a constant shifting of position in and out of the center court.

The non-thinking strategy suggests returning to the center-court position after each shot as quickly as possible, or maintaining this position until moving for a ball forces you out. At the same time, continue to hit defensive shots away from the midline of the court to keep your opponent out of this strategic court area.

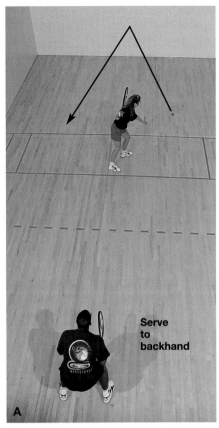

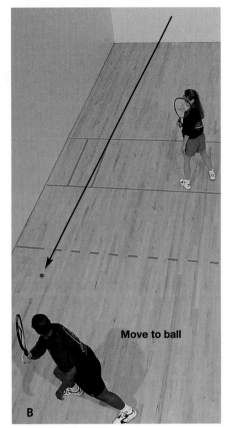

Figure 8.7 Moving directly to the ball.

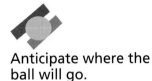

Anticipate where the ball will go.

Move to the Ball

The reason you can move your opponent out of a center-court position is simply that this player must leave center court to *play the ball*. Unfortunately, many beginning players are content to hit the ball if it is within arm's reach, regardless of where the ball is in relation to their body. This means using unorthodox strokes, few of which a player has practiced. Returns hit in this way will only rebound the ball to the front wall rather than place it. This tactic keeps the ball in play but provides neither an offensive nor a defensive advantage. You have practiced hitting forehand and backhand shots. Why not use them? The key to success in racquetball is not only knowing where to hit the ball to keep your opponent at a disadvantage, but also being able to do it. Using tried-and-true strokes will produce better game results than a contrived, over-the-shoulder punch.

To hit the ball with the same stroke requires that you move to a court position where you can make the best contact with the ball. Usually, this strategy involves playing balls off the back wall to allow the ball to drop from shoulder height as it moves through the court to a lower position off the back wall rebound. Low balls can be hit with the same forehand and backhand strokes by bending your knees and dropping your waist closer to the ground. The stroking technique remains the same.

Instead of waiting for the ball to drop from an overhead position to within arm's reach, many beginning players jump to reach the ball. Jumping is never advised as a means of getting to the ball for three reasons. First, all balls eventually will fall to the floor and could be hit from waist level. Second, jumping for the ball prevents you from stepping into the stroke and generating more power in the swing. Third, the jumping is another factor that must be controlled to hit a good return.

Therefore, jumping is neither necessary nor practical as a means of moving to the ball. This is one situation where you must wait for the ball to come to you.

Finally, when adjusting your court position to move to the ball for the best hit, it is important to move where the ball will be rather than to chase the ball around the court. Always take the shortest and most direct path to the ball's rebound (see Figure 8.7). If you find this hard to do, spend some time in a court alone, hitting the ball at various angles into the front wall, and watch the ball's movement. Beginning players who have not played a court game before must learn the rebound angles and movement of the ball through experience.

Play the Defensive Game

In summary, playing the defensive game does not mean that the beginning player should never hit an offensive shot. Rather, this strategy tries to simplify the game by minimizing the options available to the player. To some extent, these options already are minimized by the

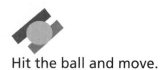

Hit the ball and move.

skill of the player and the type of shot available. If an offensive shot can be made successfully, by all means use it to end the rally. The beginning player, however, usually must concentrate on merely staying in the game and keeping the ball in play, especially with a more experienced opponent. The defensive game is designed to do this.

In general, the defensive game relies only on your ability to hit a defensive shot and keep your opponent away from the offensive center-court position. This means consistently hitting high lobs, high-Z balls, or three-wall shots to a back corner while maintaining the center-court position yourself. In this type of game, *you do not win the game as much as the opponent loses it.* Regardless, you are still the victor. This is a non-thinking strategy because your return to the front wall is predetermined before the ball leaves your racquet: a defensive shot to the opponent's backhand corner.

The other part of the non-thinking strategy is your court position. Except for the time when you are moving to hit the ball, always station yourself in the offensive center-court position. This means that as soon as the ball leaves your racquet and you can move without interfering with your opponent, return (if necessary) to the center-court position. Too often, a beginning player hits

the ball and remains stationary, waiting to see where the opponent will hit the ball. If you are positioned on one side of the court or in the front or back court, you are giving away part of the court. A ball hit to the opposite side, short or long, would be almost impossible to return. Therefore, hit the ball and *move.* Where? To the center court.

This strategy is practical not only for the beginner but also for any player who is facing a stronger, quicker, and perhaps more skilled opponent. The defensive game takes away the opponent's offensive opportunities and slows the tempo of the game. If you are not able to move fast enough to position yourself for good returns, hitting a defensive return will help to slow the ball's movement and provide more time to get in position for the next shot.

Women can find a defensive game especially effective against men. Usually men are stronger and faster and hit the ball with more power. Forcing the man to always return off slower-moving defensive shots will minimize this advantage. In addition, the defensive shot will give you some breathing room—time to reposition yourself in the center court and catch your breath.

Points to Remember

→ Begin on the offensive with your best serve, or at least with a serve that will prevent your opponent from hitting an offensive return.

→ After the serve, move to the center-court position, and return to it after each hit.

→ Hit defensive shots on all your returns, and preferably to the opponent's weak side (usually backhand).

→ Realize that defensive shots can slow down the game and help to maintain the playing tempo at a speed at which you can compete successfully.

→ Use offensive shots only if they are sure winners. Otherwise you are giving away a point.

?????

Self Testing Questions

Answers to Self Testing Questions are located on page 131.

1. After hitting a return, the beginning player should
   a. return to the center court.
   b. wait until the opponent returns the ball and move quickly to that position.
   c. move to the front court to take away an easily hit ball to the front wall.
   d. move to the back court to await a defensive return.

2. The "non-thinking" defensive strategy is good for the player who is
   a. just beginning to play racquetball.
   b. playing a more experienced opponent.
   c. playing a stronger opponent who hits harder and moves faster.
   d. all of the above.

3. Never take your eyes off the ball when it is your turn to play.　　T　　F

4. Typically, during a rally, more balls travel through the center court than any other part of the court.　　T　　F

5. Most points scored by a beginning player are the result of hitting a winning shot.　　T　　F

6. A good serving strategy is to hit your best serve to your opponent's forehand.　　T　　F

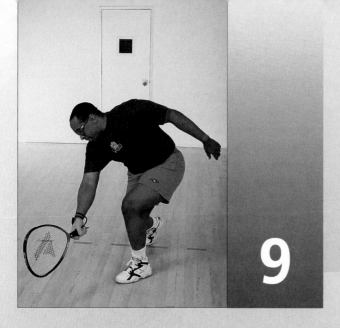

Putting the Strokes Together: Thinking Strategy

The non-thinking strategy of the defensive game becomes ineffective as a player's skills improve. When a player is able to add offensive strokes to his/her game with a predictable outcome, a thinking strategy must be used. The strategy in this type of game not only involves keeping the opponent out of an offensive court position, but also takes advantage of the opponent's weaknesses in skill or court position through ball placement and shot selection.

During this game, shots are varied but purposeful. This is a thinking strategy that calls for the player to use a variety of defensive and offensive shots. Thus, points are won rather than lost, and the style of play is more aggressive. How successful a thinking/offensive strategy can be depends upon the skill level of the players.

How to Choose the Right Serve

Minimally, the **"right"** serve is one in which an offensive shot is not returned. Ideally, the right serve results in no return to the front wall or in such a weak return that the server can hit a winning shot immediately. Which serve will be most effective in achieving these goals will vary from opponent to opponent.

It is always a good strategy to begin by hitting your best serve to your opponent's backhand. Even if a backhand serve is anticipated, the skill of your serve should score a point. Relying continually on this serve, however, will only give your opponent an opportunity to practice returning it! Variety in your serves will be the ultimate key to success at this level of play.

How can you add variety to the serve? Changing the speed of the serve, the height to the front wall, the rebound angle to the back court, or the depth to which the ball is hit in the court (Figure 9.1) will all give your serve a new look. The same basic serve can be hit to either side, short or long, high or low, hard or slow. In general, low, hard-hit serves (such as the drive and the low Z) are more effective in forcing a poor return; however, this type of serve is more difficult to control. High, softer serves (such as the lob, high Z, and garbage serve) are not as difficult to hit and, because of their placement, result in a ceiling shot return rather than an offensive shot.

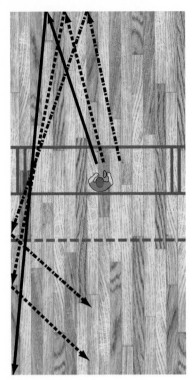

Figure 9.1 Different angles of serve and rebound depth.

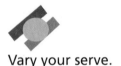

Vary your serve.

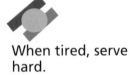

When tired, serve hard.

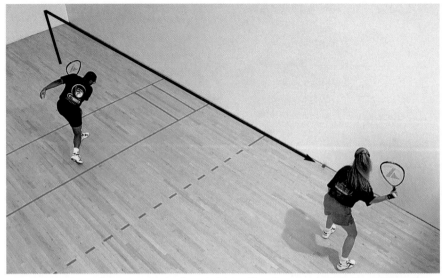

Figure 9.2 Short drive serve to forehand side, wide of center and close to side wall.

Choosing the most effective serve for the game situation varies from service to service and depends on how well you are playing. If the strengths of your game outnumber the strengths of your opponent, you can play your hard serve (drive, low Z) knowing that your skill should win the point. If the opponent's strengths outnumber yours, you need to play to a weakness and serve for a defensive return. Continue to keep your opponent on the defensive until an offensive opportunity opens for you. The type of serve you choose will set the tone for your game strategy: Attack and try to outgun your opponent, or play a more conservative game that keeps the opponent off the offensive.

You also may serve effectively to your opponent's forehand. Many players practice serving only to the backhand side. Serving only to this side of the court will take away some of the variety in your serve and allow your opponent to anticipate where the ball will be directed.

A serve to the forehand side can be effective if it is hit properly, is wide of center, and close to the side wall (see Figure 9.2). If this is your opponent's strong stroke, do not serve a hard-hit ball to the forehand court. Rather, use a lob or high-Z serve to force a defensive return. If your opponent does not have a strong forehand shot, a low drive serve usually will force a down-the-line return

on the same side of the court. If you anticipate this return and position yourself a step closer to the side wall, your second shot of the rally can be a winner. A serve also can be effective if the return of that serve sets you up for an offensive shot, regardless of how well the return of serve is hit.

Another strategy suggests: When you are tired, hit your hardest serves. Assuming that you are not the player in worse shape, your feeling of fatigue undoubtedly will be matched by your opponent. The harder the serve, the faster it must be reacted to. A tired player reacts slower or returns the ball with less power than a fresh opponent. Take advantage of your ability to control the tempo of the game by serving hard and keeping up the pressure. This would be an excellent time to hit a short drive serve if your opponent is playing deep in the back court.

With the serve, you control the game. It is the only time during play when you determine where the ball will be when you hit it. Use this advantage to set the tempo of the game, emphasize your strong skills, and force your opponent to rely on his/her weaknesses. At the very least, if a point is not won with the serve, you must be sure it is not lost because of a poorly placed serve.

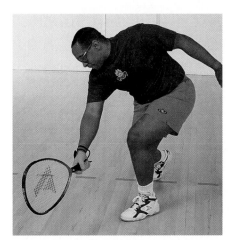

Figure 9.3 Racquet angle indicating a return to a front corner.

Listen and watch the hit.

Anticipate Your Opponent's Shot

The beginning player is restricted to playing from a center-court position during a rally because of his/her inability to *anticipate ball movement* and lack of playing skill. Most shots can be hit easily from the center court, and most poorly placed balls rebound to this area. Therefore, it is an ideal location for the novice player. The experienced player, however, usually is facing an opponent whose shot selection is varied, and ball control allows more skill in court placement. Rather than playing the court, as the beginning player does, the more experienced player plays the shot. This means you should anticipate the best return your opponent can hit and begin moving for the ball's predicted path before it is hit.

Anticipating a shot is not always guesswork. Many players will signal the kind of shot they are going to make merely by their body position relative to the ball. Because you are watching the ball at all times, you can simultaneously watch your opponent set up to hit the ball. Notice changes in stance (hip and foot placement), and racquet head angle. Look for any body or racquet position that is consistent with one particular shot (see Figure 9.3). If nothing is apparent but you are beaten continually by one particular return, use the game situation and court position as a guide as to when that shot will be used, then move to cover it.

To help anticipate the ball's movement, especially how hard the ball is hit, use your ears as well as your eyes. The sound of the ball hitting the racquet can give you a clue as to the power of the stroke. A strong hit will make a louder sound against the strings of the racquet than an easy return or a mis-hit. Listen to the sound of the hit to anticipate how hard and fast the ball will rebound off the front wall.

Use the Court Wisely

A player's **court position** can be used to an advantage in two ways. One is to take away the opponent's best shot—the shot that has a high probability of being a winner—and the second is to keep your opponent moving in the court with the purpose of tiring out this player.

The first use of the court requires that you maintain a court position to either (1) make your opponent's best return shot impossible to hit or (2) place you in the ideal position to hit the ball off this return. This tactic is important only when your opponent has been successful in scoring consistently off one return. To prevent losing more points to this shot, you must position yourself to make this shot ineffective. An example would be staying to the left of center to discourage a down-the-line shot in order to force a weaker cross-court return.

To be effective, your court position must be fixed before the opponent returns the ball. Otherwise your court position has not helped you. The purpose of positioning yourself on the court in this manner is to eliminate this shot as one of your opponent's options.

The objective of the second use of the court is to literally keep your opponent running. Shot selection is determined not only by the other player's weaknesses but also with consideration as to how far your opponent would have to move to get to the ball. For example, if you have just hit the ball to the backhand side, return the ball to the forehand side. Varying placement of the ball short and long is also effective if your opponent has not anticipated the short ball and set up for this return. Even the most conditioned player will fatigue after long rallies in which the ball must be hit from all parts of the court. This tactic can be especially valuable at the end of the game when fatigue causes slower reaction and movement times.

Return to the Offensive Position

Since the serve provides the server with the first opportunity to score, the server is considered to be the offensive player. As such, the server is initially in control of the game. Thus, it is the job of the receiver to regain the serve and thus the offense. The first step in this strategy requires that you move the opponent out of the center-court position. Any of the defensive strokes or a down-the-line or cross-court return will work equally well. The preference for the latter two shots is that they are offensive returns and have the potential for ending the rally immediately. Neither of these strokes, however, should be hit unless the ball is served at knee level or below. Balls that are served high off the front wall or that rebound high into the back court (lob, Z ball, ceiling) should be hit with your best defensive return. With any of these returns, the server will be pulled out of the center-court position, which you now can assume. Consequently, you have eliminated the server's offensive court advantage and regained this position yourself.

To make the best return off serves that rebound off the floor high against the back wall, make it a practice to hit the serves as soon after the floor bounce as possible. If you allow the ball to strike the back wall, you must hit the ball as it falls to the floor, possibly very close to the corner. Hitting the serve before it touches the back wall usually will give you a better shot opportunity. Similarly, balls that would run the corner should be taken before the corner is hit. Otherwise, you will face a very difficult return. This may mean positioning yourself a step or two closer to the front wall and away from the back wall to catch the bounce.

Returning to the offensive can be done in two ways: (1) hit a winning shot off the return (kill or passing shot), or (2) hit a defensive shot that forces the server to leave the center-court position. The choice of the return usually depends on the choice of serve. A low ball (below your knees) is a prime candidate for an offensive return; a high ball above your shoulder, a defensive shot. Balls falling in between either should be taken before dropping below shoulder level or hit after falling below the knee. Balls that rebound off the floor to the back wall should be taken after the floor bounce.

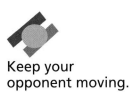

Keep your opponent moving.

Hit a Winning Shot

A shot can result in a score for one of three reasons: (1) the ball was hit so well that the opponent could not return it even though in proper court position (kill shot); (2) the ball was hit to an area of the court that the opponent could not reach in time to return the ball (passing shot); or (3) the opponent just missed the ball—an unforced error. The third reason for a score may be related to your play only if you had hit for long rallies consistently with defensive shots to tire out the opposing player. Otherwise, unforced errors must be considered as resulting from a mental lapse on your opponent's part, and you cannot take credit for the point.

The first and second reasons for a winning shot depend upon your play. To hit a winning shot, you must be aggressive. Always move quickly to the ball, and align yourself correctly for the proper hit. Never wait for the ball to come to you or be satisfied with hitting the ball if it happens to be within reach if you can maneuver for a better shot.

There are three times when you can consider hitting the ball as it rebounds from the front wall (see Chapter 4). Which you choose depends on how aggressively you are playing and whether you want to speed up or slow down the game. The first is after the ball comes off the front wall and before it hits the floor. Hitting a volley is effective for speeding up play and possibly catching your opponent out of court position. The best return for a winning shot off a volley is a cross-court or a down-the-line passing shot. Care must be taken, however, not to hit the pass so hard that the ball rebounds off the back wall into the center-court playing area.

If you choose to let the ball bounce, it may be hit immediately after touching the floor as it passes between your shoelaces and knee, or finally after the height of the arc is reached and the ball is falling to the floor, passing again through this same area. Aggressive players try to take most balls on the skip, just after the floor is hit. This also works to speed up play and may catch the opponent out of court position. In addition, it offers the advantage of being at the right position from which to hit a kill shot.

Waiting until the ball arcs and is falling for the second time to the floor gives you more time to set up for the shot, and your opponent more time to set up for the return. Therefore, hitting the ball at this point should be done primarily by the beginning player who reacts slowly to the ball, or by the experienced player who is trying to slow down the game.

Regardless of where you are when you hit the ball or what kind of ball you hit, move to cut off your opponent's anticipated return after you hit the ball. There you will be the least vulnerable to your opponent's next shot, and you can begin to set up for another winning return.

A Good Defense May Be the Best Offense

Every player will meet someone who is a match against the best serves or who can anticipate the ball's movement in the court and can score at will. Often this occurs when a beginning player plays a more experienced player., As a result, because of the speed and power of his or her strokes, the more experienced player seems to be playing in a different time zone.

The only way to make a game of this situation is to try to outmaneuver the power. This can be done in three ways: (1) slow the ball and the tempo of the game by waiting to hit the ball just before the second bounce; (2) use defensive return shots to the opponent's weak side and hit garbage serves; and (3) keep your opponent out of the center court by hitting balls wide of the midline. Trying to outgun power usually leads to a sloppy game, referred to as Battleball (see Chapter 7). Using a strategy that never gives your opponent anything good to hit or a court position from which to hit it eliminates power as a factor.

Thus, the best offense for some experienced players against a power player is a good defensive game. It may

not have the spark and strong rallies of a power game, but the weaker player who is the tactician will have a chance to score.

This is not to imply that the player can never hit offensive shots but, rather, that these shots should be attempted only when there is a high probability of success. Indeed, the defensive game should be used to tire out the opponent by moving him/her around the court, frustrating him/her into an unforced error, or soliciting a weak return that sets up your offensive shot. The name of this game is patience—patience to endure the long rallies and wait for your opening to an offensive position. Above all, to use this strategy effectively, you must be careful never to hit a low ball to your opponent's strong side, because that is just the opportunity needed to begin a power game.

Play the Weakness

Every player has a weakness—a shot the player would prefer not to hit. Your job is to find that weakness and take advantage of it if you can. If the opponent does not appear to have a weakness, create one through ball placement and court position. A player who is running to hit a ball constantly will fatigue no matter how well conditioned, so keep the ball moving. If the player is much stronger than you, go for broke. Try to hit everything and anything, even the best kill shot. If you concede the shot, the point is lost; if you try for the ball, you may return just a few and stop a rally. If nothing else, Mr./Ms. Sharpshooter may think twice about the choice of hits, knowing that you came close to returning a ball. This hesitancy may cause some mis-hits and provide better opportunities for making offensive returns.

To have any hope that this strategy will succeed, give yourself the best chance for hitting a winner. Never hit the ball and hold court position. *Move* to cut off the return, and *hustle*. If this strategy doesn't work, at least you put up a fight!

The best offense may be a good defense.

Points to Remember

→ Play an offensive game, plan your shots, and move your opponent around the court to set up your best return.

→ Vary your serves by changing the force of the hit, the angle off the front wall, and where the ball rebounds behind the short line.

→ Anticipate your opponent's shot, and move to a court position to block it or set up for the return.

→ Use defensive shots from the back-court position and offensive returns from a center- or front-court position.

→ Keep your opponent away from a center-court position by hitting the ball wide of the midline of the court and into the back corners.

→ When you are tired, hit harder and move faster.

→ When playing a stronger opponent, play a defensive game and slow the tempo of play.

→ When playing doubles, communicate with your partner and decide how to divide up court coverage before play begins.

Thinking Strategy for Doubles

Because of the number of players on the court during a game of doubles, there is more opportunity for injury than when playing a single opponent. Consequently, with four players on a small court at the same time, it is important that all players are *thinking* during play! Running into an opponent or your partner, striking another player instead of the ball, or two players going for the same shot will occur when players consider only the ball and not the other participants on the court. Thus, to play doubles successfully you must not only *think* while you play, but communicate with your partner about playing strategy as well.

The first decision you and your partner must make is how you will work together to cover the court. There are three basic ways to share court responsibility. The first, and most basic, is simply to divide the court in half lengthwise and play side by side. One player will take all balls landing on the right side of the court (Figure 9.4), while his/her partner takes balls landing on the left side of the court. In this court strategy, each player must cover his or her side of the

court regardless of where the ball touches the floor in relation to the front wall. The key to the successful use of this positioning is to (1) assign the best player to take backhand shots and, (2) predetermine who will take balls rebounding down the middle of the court. This prevents both players "courteously" allowing his/her partner the opportunity to take the middle-court shot and end up with neither player reacting to the ball. If a team has both a right-handed and left-handed player, make sure that the players set up on the court so that their forehand strokes are toward the nearest wall. The player with the best backhand should then be assigned to take balls that rebound down the middle of the court.

This position strategy is good to use for beginning players and for players that are approximately equal in playing ability. It allows each player to focus on a well-defined area of the court and concentrate on hitting the ball. This strategy also minimizes spontaneous decision-making and conflict between partners.

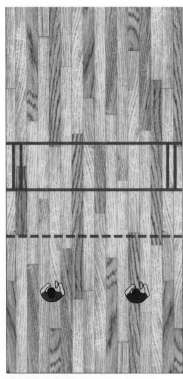

Figure 9.4 Playing side by side.

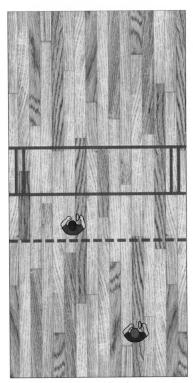

Figure 9.5 Up and back coverage.

The second court position strategy is to again divide the court in half, but this time the division identifies a front court and a back court coverage, commonly referred to as "up and back" (see Figure 9.5). In this strategy, one partner is positioned by the short line and the other is an arm's length away from the back wall. Both players cover their area of the court from side wall to side wall. This strategy is good for players that bring different playing strengths to the court. In particular, if one player is skilled in offensive kill shots, he or she should be the "up" player. If a player is particularly good at hitting defensive shots or taking shots that rebound off the back corners of the court, he/she should cover the back position. Another way to decide who plays "up" is based on speed of movement. Good front-court play is best accomplished by players that are quick and agile. This is because the front player not only has to respond to opponents' kill shots from this position, but also when receiving the serve, must quickly readjust from a service return court position (i.e., back court) to the service-court area. If these qualities are not present in either player, then an "up and back" strategy of court coverage is not advised. If both players have equal strengths in both offensive and defensive returns and movement on the court, they can alternate the "up and back" positions. This can be done simply by predetermining that the partner not returning the serve will move to a forward-court position. The partner returning the serve will protect the back-court area.

The third strategy for court coverage divides the court into two triangles. The triangles are determined by a diagonal boundary extending from the short line/side wall intersection to the opposite side wall/back wall juncture. Whether the diagonal is "drawn" toward the back right or left corner of the court depends on the preference of the partners (Figure 9.6), and which partner wants to cover the front- vs. the back-court area. The fastest (offensive) player should cover the short line and a very little of the back court. The defensive player should defend the back-court area and balls that rebound along the side wall within his or her triangle. Again, there must be discussion between the two partners to determine who will play balls rebounding along the diagonal. Make this decision before starting play! The side wall that each player "protects" is determined in the same way as the side-by-side strategy. Keep the player with the strongest backhand on the left side of the court or, in the case of a right-handed/left-handed pairing, place the players' forehands toward the nearest wall. This strategy should be used for players more experienced with the game, since it requires an awareness of where balls will rebound to determine which partner should take the shot. However, it can also be effective for players of significantly different skill levels, with the more highly skilled player always covering the front position along with the back corner, and the less skilled player taking primarily defensive shots along the back wall.

Regardless of which court strategy you choose to use, when playing doubles it is important during play to

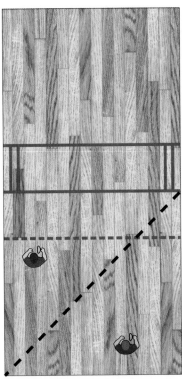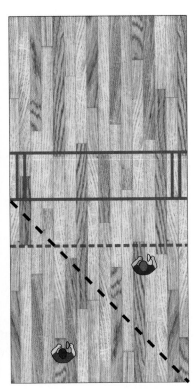

Figure 9.6 Diagonal court coverage.

communicate with your partner. Unless your partner is a mind reader, talking to each other when it is your turn to hit the ball ensures that you are aware of each other's position and intent. This is critical to ensure safe and successful play. Obviously, it is not courteous to discuss your play during your opponent's return unless you want a yelling match on court!

Since the game of cut-throat places a single player against a doubles team, these strategies are also useful when playing with a partner during cut-throat competition. However, because you will be playing with two different partners during this game, communication about court coverage is especially important before each point.

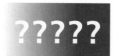

Self Testing Questions

Answers to Self Testing Questions are located on page 131.

1. In order to maintain an offensive center-court position, you can
   a. return the ball wide of center.
   b. hit a high rebound into the back court.
   c. hit a down-the-line shot.
   d. all of the above.

2. Your best chance of winning occurs if you
   a. hustle.
   b. anticipate your opponent's shot.
   c. play to your opponent's weakness.
   d. all of the above.

3. While the beginning player plays the court, the experienced player plays and anticipates the shot.   T   F

4. Kill shots should be hit from balls that have dropped below the knee.   T   F

5. When playing a more experienced opponent, stay in the front court to protect against kill shots.   T   F

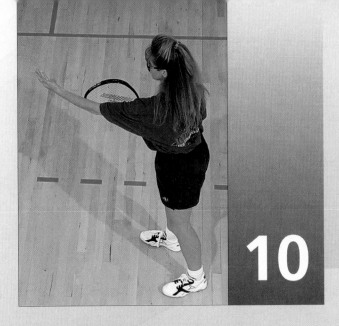

10

Drills for the Player

Racquetball drills are useful in helping the beginning player develop the skills necessary to play the game and in giving the experienced player opportunity to practice and sharpen all shots. Drills may also be used as part of your warm-up routine to help you get the feel for the court and the ball's movement, as well as help to adjust your body to exercise.

The following list of drills was designed to provide the player with an opportunity to work on the strokes and shots used most often in a game situation. Evaluative measures accompany some drills to help you determine your proficiency with that skill and when you will be ready to incorporate it into your game plan.

The drills are listed from the most basic skills to playing modified games with an opponent. The beginning player can either start with the first drill and work through to the simulated games, or pick the drills that work on the skills that are most difficult.

In all drills, starting the ball in play is critical. The ball can be either dropped to the floor or tossed against a wall. When dropped, you must be sure to drop the ball in front of your forward foot so you can step into the stroke

when contacting the ball. If the ball is tossed to a wall, position yourself so the rebound falls in front of your body position. This will allow you to step forward to meet the ball. The wrong ball toss will result in learning to stroke at a ball that is positioned improperly in relation to your body.

Scoring Scales

Scoring scales are presented in selected drills. The illustrations accompanying these drills indicate the size of the target area (1' or 2') and the points allotted to each target zone (5, 3, or 1). Balls in the targeted area can be scored by making a best guess or by placing small pieces of masking tape on the floor and walls to outline the areas. Balls that hit a line between two point areas should be given the lower of the two scores. A legal shot not hitting the target area is scored 0 points. Although the target points are somewhat arbitrary, they do identify, through points scored, the accuracy and placement of your shots. In general, the percentages listed in the table on the following page can be used to determine the effectiveness of your returns and serves.

CATEGORY	PERCENT	USE
Excellent	90 – 100	"bread and butter" shot; use this shot whenever your strategy dictates
Good	75 – 89	consistent enough to use to vary your shots; a dependable shot in a game in which you are in control
Average	50 – 74	Be careful—you may miss this shot half of the time; not the shot to choose when the game is close, but a good shot to practice when you can afford to lose some points
Below Average	below 50	POISON!—do not hit this in a game situation because you will miss it more than half of the time

DRILL I
WATCHING THE GAME

Purpose: To develop a concept of how racquetball is played and the use of offensive and defensive shots during the game.

Method: Go to a court with an observation area, and watch experienced players play racquetball. Count the number of offensive and defensive shots used by each player.

DRILL II
FOREHAND SHOTS

Purpose: To practice hitting a forehand shot to the back corners of the court from three primary areas of the floor.

Method: Hit eight balls each from the mid-, center-, and back-court positions. From each position, hit four balls to the back right corner and four balls to the back left corner. Hit the ball after you've dropped it to the floor.

DRILL III
BACKHAND SHOTS

Purpose: To practice hitting a backhand shot to the back corners of the court from three primary areas of the floor.

Method: Hit eight balls each from the mid-, center-, and back-court positions. From each position, hit four balls to the back right corner and four balls to the back left corner. Hit the ball after you've dropped it to the floor.

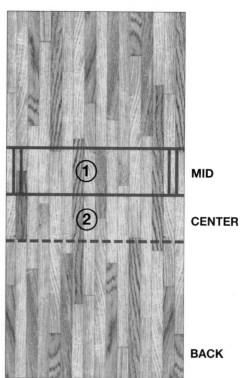

Hitting positions for stroking drill.

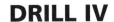

DRILL IV
FOREHAND AND BACKHAND SHOTS FROM SIDE-WALL TOSS

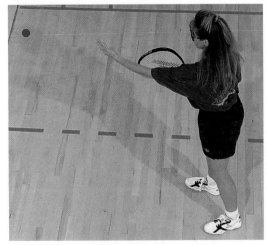

Purpose: To practice hitting forehand and backhand shots to the back corners of the court from a ball bouncing off the side wall.

Method: Stand with your hips pivoted and facing the side wall appropriate for either a forehand or backhand stroke. Toss the ball into the side wall. After the rebound, hit the ball to a back corner of the court. Hit eight balls from each of the three court positions, four to each corner, then repeat eight shots each from the same court positions with the other stroke.

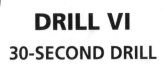
Toss off the side wall.

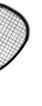

DRILL V
SUICIDE DRILL

Purpose: To develop muscular endurance and anaerobic capacity, and to practice moving to the ball and returning it to the front wall.

Method: Begin in the center court, and after dropping the ball, hit it to the front wall. Continue to return the ball as quickly as you can, hitting all balls regardless of their court position or the number of times the ball has bounced off the floor. Work at positioning yourself correctly for each hit. Continue this drill for 2-minute intervals, allowing yourself to rest 30 seconds to 1 minute after each hitting session. Repeat the drill 10 times. Record the number of balls hit each 2-minute interval.

DRILL VI
30-SECOND DRILL

Purpose: To teach the player to react quickly to the ball's court position and improve his/her movement time, and to work on ball control.

Method: Begin in a center-court position. Drop the ball and return it to the front wall. Continue to return the ball off the rebound, counting the number of times the ball is returned in 30 seconds. Count only the shots that would be legal returns in a game. Do this drill at least every other practice session. Try to improve one to three shots each time.

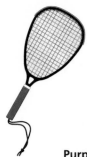

DRILL VII
SERVING DRILL—LOB AND HIGH Z

Purpose: To practice hitting lob and high Z serves correctly and accurately to a back-corner court position.

Method: Standing close to the center of the service zone, hit 10 lob serves to the right back corner of the court to the designated target area. Score each serve as indicated in the diagram. Give one point to a legal serve if it lands on the correct side of the court but not into the back corner. Total the points. Refer to the scoring scale to determine the accuracy of this serve. Total points possible = 50 points. Repeat this drill with the lob serve to the left back corner and the target area. Score and evaluate. Total points = 50. (Note: for a lob hit with a backhand stroke, you may move in the service area toward the backhand side wall.) Repeat both parts of this drill using a high-Z serve. Total points possible for each part = 50 points.

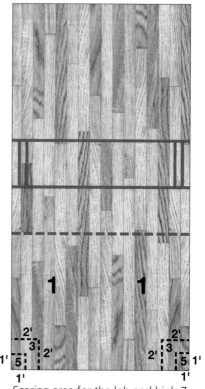

Scoring area for the lob and high-Z serving drill.

SCORING SCALE:	
	Points
Excellent	45–50
Good	39–44
Average	25–38
Below Average	fewer than 25

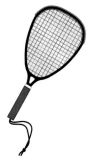

DRILL VIII

SERVING DRILLS—DRIVE SERVE

Purpose: To develop accuracy in your drive serve and be able to drive serve to a variety of court positions.

Method: From the center of the service zone, hit three drive serves to each of the four designated court positions. Repeat the circuit three times. Score one point for each correct placement. Total points possible = 36. (Note: you can total points scored to each designated area to indicate your most accurate placement. Total points to each area = 9.)

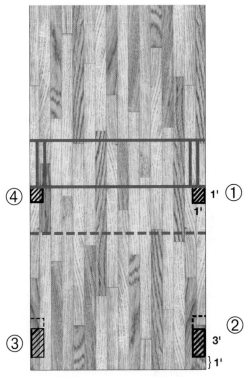

Scoring area for the drive serve.

SCORING SCALE:

	Points
Excellent	32–36
Good	27–31
Average	18–26
Below Average	fewer than 18

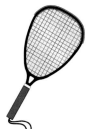

DRILL IX

DEFENSIVE SHOTS—LOB, CEILING, HIGH Z, AROUND-THE-WALL

Purpose: To practice hitting a defensive shot from two court positions and develop accuracy in ball placement.

Method: Using a dropped ball, hit each defensive shot 10 times, from center- and back-court positions (five to each corner). Use the same target area as designated for the lob and high-Z serves. Total points possible for each serve from each position = 50. To vary this drill, begin the defensive shot with a side-wall toss.

SCORING SCALE:

	Points
Excellent	45–50
Good	39–44
Average	25–38
Below Average	fewer than 25

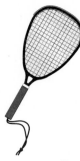

DRILL X
BACK WALL DRILL

Purpose: To practice hitting balls rebounding off the back wall and accurately returning them wide of the midline in a back-court area.

Method: Standing in the back court, toss balls into the back wall to rebound for a forehand stroke. Hit 10 balls, returning each to the front. Score the rebound in the designated area. Total points possible = 50. Repeat the drill using a ball toss to your backhand side, and return the balls with a backhand stroke. Total points possible = 50.

SCORING SCALE:	
	Points
Excellent	45–50
Good	39–44
Average	25–38
Below Average	fewer than 25

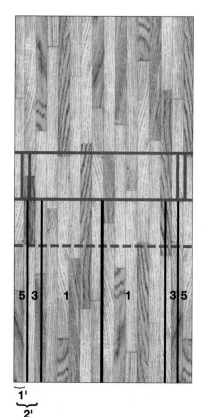

Scoring area for the back wall drill.

DRILL XI
CORNER RETURN

Purpose: To practice hitting balls after they have rebounded from a back corner and accurately returning them into a back-court position wide of the midline.

Method: Standing in the back court, toss a ball to your forehand side to rebound either from the back wall to a side wall or in the opposite direction. Return 10 balls with your forehand stroke, then turn and toss 10 balls to the opposite side/back wall for a backhand return. Hit each ball to rebound into a back-court position and wide of the midline of the court. Score each return with the same designated target area used for the back-wall returns. Total points possible for each stroke = 50.

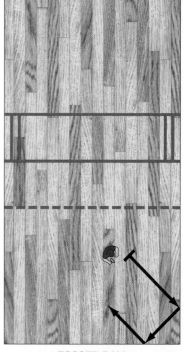

Path of a tossed ball for the corner hit drill—side wall toss.

TOSSED BALL

SCORING SCALE:

	Points
Excellent	45–50
Good	39–44
Average	25–38
Below Average	fewer than 25

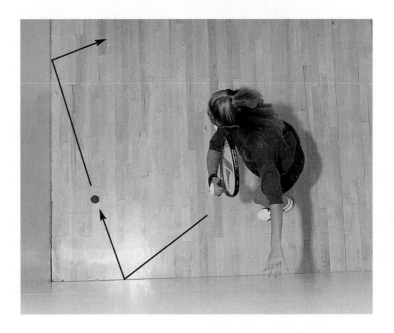

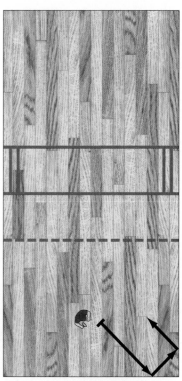

TOSSED BALL

Path of a tossed ball for the corner hit drill—back wall toss.

DRILL XII
REPEAT CEILING SHOTS

Purpose: To practice hitting balls rebounding off the back wall and accurately returning them wide of the midline in a back-court area.

Method: Standing in the back court, toss balls into the back wall to rebound for a forehand stroke. Hit 10 balls, returning each to the front. Score the rebound in the designated area. Total points possible = 50. Repeat the drill using a ball toss to your backhand side, and return the balls with a backhand stroke. Total points possible = 50.

SCORING SCALE:	
	Points
Excellent	45–50
Good	39–44
Average	25–38
Below Average	fewer than 25

DRILL XIII
OFFENSIVE SHOTS—PASSING

Purpose: To practice hitting passing shots from two court positions and accurately directing them to one of two court areas.

Method: Using a side-wall toss to your forehand side, hit 10 passing shots from court positions A and B. Return the ball into the shaded area of the court diagram. Score one point for each successful return. Total points possible = 10. Repeat the drill using a backhand stroke. Total points possible = 10.

SCORING SCALE:	
	Points
Excellent	9–10
Good	7–8
Average	5–6
Below Average	fewer than 5

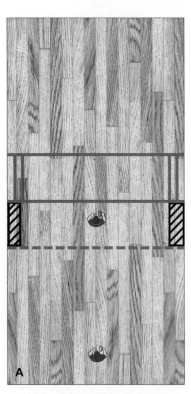

Target area for a passing shot from a back court position.

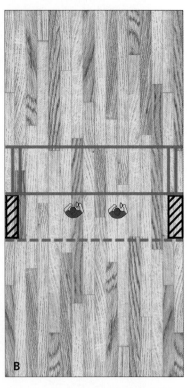

Target area for a passing shot from a center court position.

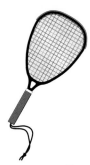

DRILL XIV
OFFENSIVE SHOTS—KILL

Purpose: To practice hitting accurate kill shots from three court positions.

Method: Dropping the ball to your forehand side, hit 10 kill shots from each court position: A, B, and C. Score each position separately using a front-wall target area. Use corner and pinch kill shots. Total points possible = 50. Repeat the drill using a drop to your backhand side. Total points possible = 50 from each court position. This drill can also be varied by using a side-wall toss to put the ball in play.

SCORING SCALE:

	Points
Excellent	45–50
Good	39–44
Average	25–38
Below Average	fewer than 25

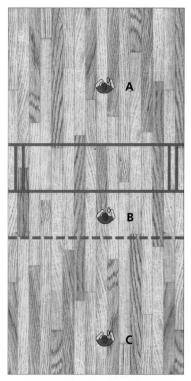

Hitting positions for the kill shot drill.

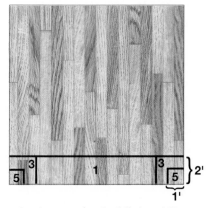

Scoring area for the kill shot drill.

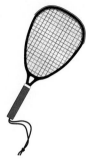

DRILL XV
RALLY DRILL—HIT AND MOVE

Purpose: To practice hitting a ball and moving away from the rebound to avoid colliding with your opponent on the court.

Method: Standing side by side in the back court with your opponent, the player on the right side of the court hits a ball straight into the front wall. After hitting, this player moves to the left and out of the way of the opponent moving toward the ball. The ball is again returned straight into the front wall, and the positions are again reversed. Continue this rotation until the ball is missed.

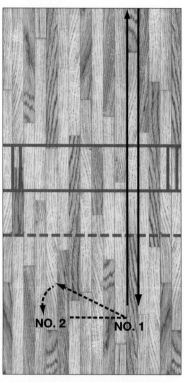

Rally drill to avoid collisions
on the court.

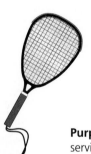

DRILL XVI
MINI-GAME

Purpose: To give players a chance to practice serving and returning the serve.

Method: Each player serves five times and then rotates to the back court to be the receiver. The game is to 15 points, and a point is scored by either player on each rally regardless of whether he/she was serving.

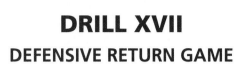

DRILL XVII
DEFENSIVE RETURN GAME

Purpose: To practice hitting a defensive shot off any serve.

Method: Only the server scores. The server must use a drive serve and the receiver a ceiling or other defensive return. If the receiver does not use this type of return, the server scores a point. If the drive serve is not hit, a side-out occurs. Variation: Change the type of serve required to be hit, or specify exactly which defensive shot is to be returned.

DRILL XVIII
GAME WARM-UP DRILL

Purpose: To provide a method for warming up before a game.

Method: Begin by standing side by side with your opponent just behind the short line. Practice hitting forehand strokes to the front wall. After several minutes, move two-thirds of the way back to the back wall and practice ceiling shots from this position. Finally, back up to the back wall and hit offensive and defensive returns to the front wall from a ball-toss off the back wall.

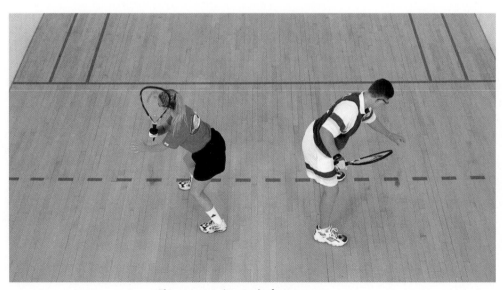

Players warming up before a game.

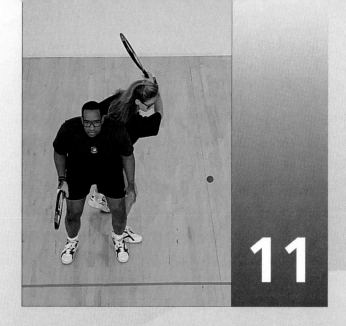

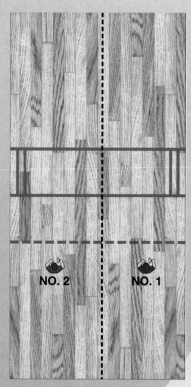

Court Etiquette and Interpreting the Rules

11

As in all sport activities, a degree of courtesy is involved in a competitive racquetball game. We need to understand and interpret the rules of the game in a fair and objective manner. With two individuals enclosed in a space of 20' x 40' x 20', there is little room for disagreement. The possibility of injury and negative feelings increases if every courtesy is not extended to the opponent and if the rules are not complied with meticulously.

Prior to the Start

Prior to the start of the match, the court must be shared by players executing the shots to be used in the match. In that warm-up, each player should control ball placement to avoid interfering with the opponent. The court should be divided in length, and all shots should be hit within that boundary (see Figures 11.1 and 11.2). During the warm-up, players should hit only shots they can control, and they should be considerate if the opponent retrieves a ball from the front of the court. Stopping execution of a shot if the opponent walks in front of you or moves to your court to retrieve a ball are specific examples (see Figure

11.3). Bouncing the ball back to the opponent is also appreciated and in good taste (see Figure 11.4).

Figure 11.1 Court divided in length for warm-up.

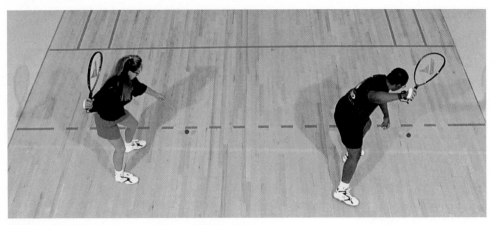

Figure 11.2 Two players warming up side by side.

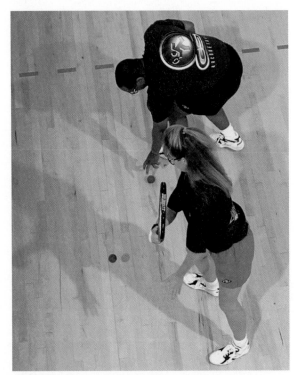

Figure 11.3 Stopping execution of warm-up shot when a player walks in front of another player.

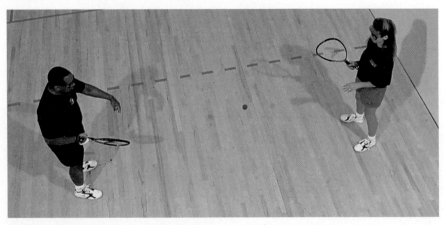

Figure 11.4 Bouncing the ball back to opponent when warming up.

About the Rally, Game and Match, Serving, and Ball in Play

Instituting proper etiquette and interpretation of the rules during the game is crucial to acceptable play. Some of the rules are quite simple, yet the beginning player sometimes does not respond initially to the obvious and has to be informed of a rule that most experienced players take for granted.

Rally, Points, and Outs

A rally occurs once the ball is placed in play by a serve, and it continues until a player fails to hit the front wall prior to the ball striking the floor, when the ball touches the floor twice, or as a result of a hinder. Points are scored (see Appendix, Rule 1.4 Points and Outs) only by the serving side at the conclusion of a rally. A serve lost following a rally is called a sideout (in singles), or handout (in doubles). The objective of racquetball is to win each rally by serving or returning serve until the opponent fails to keep the ball in play (see Appendix, Rule 1.3 Objective).

Game and Match

How to keep score is one of those rules that is taken for granted, yet should be explained. A game is won when the first player reaches 15 points; thus, a score of 15–14 is a legal game. To win a match in most situations requires you to win the best of three games. If each player has won one game, the third game is played to 11 points, again with the need

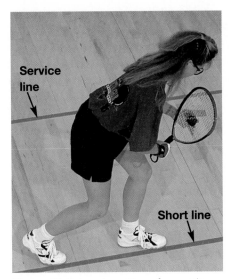

Figure 11.5 Legal position of server in relation to serving zone.

You have to win only by one point.

to win by only one point (see Rule 1.5 Match, Game, Tiebreaker). In class situations, students may discover that games are played to an assortment of final points to accommodate class procedure.

Serving

Specific *rules govern the service* in racquetball (see Appendix, Rule 3.1 Serve). Determination of who serves begins with a coin toss or, in casual play, "lagging" (select a target and the closest to hitting the target serves first) for serve. The winner of the coin toss elects to receive or serve in the first game, with the second game beginning in reverse order. If a tiebreaker is required, then the player with the most total points will have the option of serving or receiving (a tie requires another coin flip or "lag"). To begin play, the server must stand between the short line and the service line—an area commonly called the **service zone**. The service zone is defined as the back of the paint of the short line and the front of the service line paint (go back to Figure 1.1 on page 1 to check out the service zone). Any part of either foot may not fully extend

beyond either line of the service zone; however, stepping *on* the line is allowed. To initiate a serve, the player must drop the ball (Figure 11.5) and then strike it with the racquet after the ball rebounds off the floor. Following racquet contact on the serve, the ball must strike the front wall first on the fly and then carry beyond the short line. The ball must strike the floor beyond the short line before hitting the back wall, ceiling, or more than one side wall. A screen serve, an illegal drive serve, and a serve that strikes the front wall on the fly and doesn't carry beyond the short line are **fault serves**. Serves that hit two or more side walls, the back wall on the fly, and the ceiling on the fly are also fault serves. All together there are nine fault serves (see Appendix, Rule 3.9 Fault Serves). Common terms for a fault include a "short" for a serve that doesn't carry past the short line, a "long" for a ball that hits the back wall on the fly, and "two-wall" for a serve that hits more than one side wall on the fly (see Figures 11.6, 11.7, and 11.8).

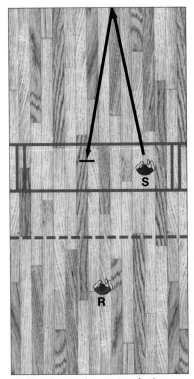

Figure 11.6 Short serve fault.

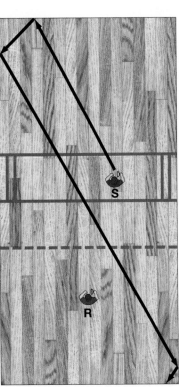

Figure 11.7 Two-wall fault.

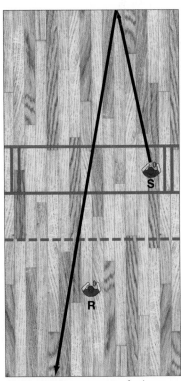

Figure 11.8 Long serve fault.

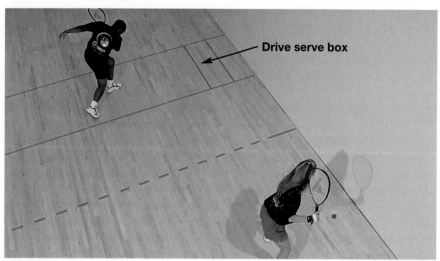

Figure 11.9 Drive serve box.

Avoid hinders:
keep moving.

The fault serve mentioned above as an illegal drive serve deserves special mention. There is a **drive serve zone** (see Appendix, Rule 3.6 Drive Service Zones) that consists of two drive serve lines, each 3 feet from the side wall, located in the service zone. The server may drive serve to the same side of the court that the serve is initiated as long as the start and finish of the server's serve motion take place outside of the 3-foot drive serve box (see Figure 11.9). A second serve opportunity is provided following all fault serves.

An **out serve** signifies the loss of serve. Loss of serve occurs when the ball does not hit the front wall on the fly after the server hits the ball, or when two faults are served in succession. There are additional out serves, including: an out-of-court serve, a missed serve attempt, a crotch serve off the front wall, a touched serve, a fake balk serve, an illegal hit, a safety zone violation with the server or doubles partner entering the zone before the serve crosses the short line, and a serve striking a partner who is standing outside the doubles box in a doubles match (see Appendix, Rule 3.10 Out Serves).

Calling the score prior to every serve is expected in a racquetball match. The server's score is always called first, alerting your opponent that both parties agree to the score unless the opponent stops play to question it. Also, calling the score implies that the next serve is going to follow shortly and the opponent should be ready to receive.

Ball in Play

Once the ball is in play, each of the players must hit it (in singles) alternately. The ultimate goal of either player is to hit the ball so it strikes the front wall before hitting the floor. A ball can hit the back wall, followed by the ceiling and side walls, as long as it eventually gets to the front wall before touching the floor.

A server continues the serve for each point played until two faults are hit in succession, an out serve is made, or the server cannot return the opponent's shot in a legal manner (that is, not returning the ball to the front wall before it strikes the floor, hitting after the second bounce, or committing a point hinder). A return-of-serve player remains in that situation until the serving opponent has made one of the above-mentioned errors.

Hinders

Hinders have to be discussed in detail when interpreting the rules. The two basic types of hinders in racquetball are: (1) **avoidable hinders**, usually intentional acts to prevent an opponent from a fair try at hitting the ball and (2) **dead-ball hinders**, (commonly-called hinders), accidental and also associated with preventing the opponent from having a fair chance at the ball.

Avoidable hinders are usually called on a player who intentionally moves in the path of an opponent to prevent the opponent from hitting the ball or seeing it clearly. Avoidable hinders penalize the offending player by a loss of the rally. Experienced players are quite skilled at committing an avoidable hinder called **blocking**. The player committing the infraction may hit a shot from an "up" position and then set up to block the movement of the opponent in a "back" position (see Figure 11.10). The movement is subtle and discourages the opponent from making an attempt to reach the ball, since the opponent is in a "back" position.

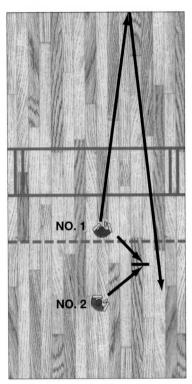

Figure 11.10 Blocking an opponent in back court: avoidable hinder.

There are countless avoidable hinders in racquetball (see Appendix, Rule 3.15, Avoidable Hinders). The player who simply will not move to permit an opponent access to the ball is one example (see Figure 11.11). A second example is a player who will move next to an opponent attempting a full-swing shot. That opponent will not be able to complete the swing because of the position of the other player (see Figure 11.12). A third example is a player pushing or shoving an opponent as a means of gaining impetus to move to reach a ball. Pushing off an opponent gives an unfair advantage, since it may place the opponent in an off-balance position for the next shot (see Figure 11.13).

A fourth distinct violation associated with avoidable hinders is the intentional moving of the body into the path of the return shot of an opponent. If an opponent strikes the ball from a "back" position and the "up" player (recognizing that the shot would put that player at a great disadvantage for a return) moves into the path of the ball, the call is an avoidable hinder (see Figure 11.14).

Dead-ball hinders occur as part of the action of the game and happen without a planned effort (see Appendix, Rule 3.14, Dead-Ball Hinders). The first example is a court hinder. A court hinder occurs when the ball strikes an irregular portion of the court, such as an edge of the door (Figure 11.15), a can placed in the corner of the court (Figure 11.16), or any other part of the court that would impede the progress of play.

Other examples of dead-ball hinders include (1) a player who is hit by an opponent's shot prior to the ball striking the front wall (Figure 11.17); (2) a ball that is "screened" so the opponent cannot see the ball clearly (Figure 11.18); and (3) a ball that goes between the legs of the opponent (Figure 11.19), distracting the player hitting the ball (not always a hinder, depending on player positioning and proximity of players).

In addition, when two players collide while attempting to move out of the way of each other or the ball (Figure 11.20) or attempting to reach the ball, play is stopped and a hinder is called. A final hinder is called any time a player about to execute a stroke believes the opponent will be placed at risk safety-wise.

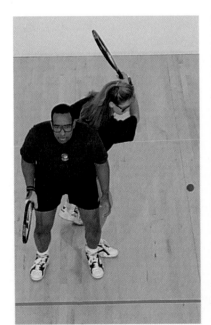

Figure 11.11 A player who doesn't move out of the way: avoidable hinder.

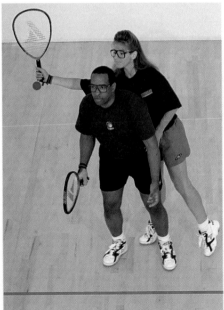

Figure 11.12 A player moving too close to a player attempting a shot: avoidable hinder.

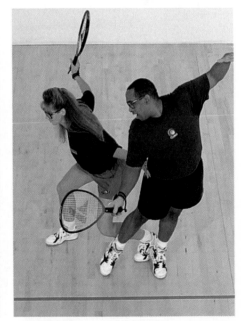

Figure 11.13 A player pushing an opponent to get a ball: avoidable hinder.

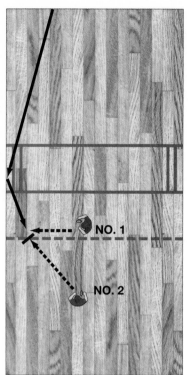

Figure 11.14 Moving into opponent's path: avoidable hinder.

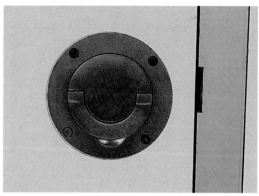

Figure 11.15 Ball hitting edge of door: dead-ball hinder.

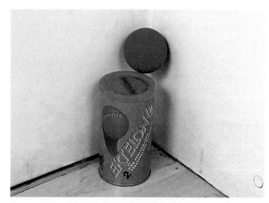

Figure 11.16 Ball hitting ball can: dead ball hinder.

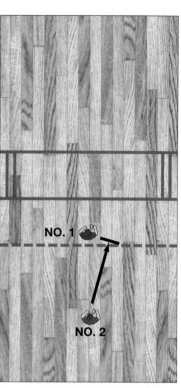

Figure 11.17 Being hit by opponent's shot: dead-ball hinder.

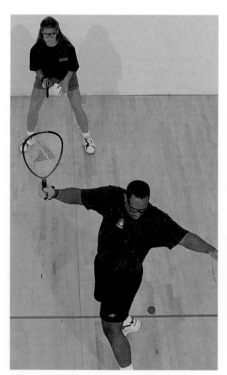

Figure 11.18 Screening the ball: dead-ball hinder.

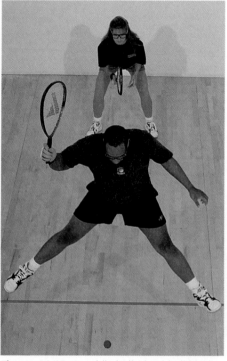

Figure 11.19 Straddle ball: dead-ball hinder when screening the opponent.

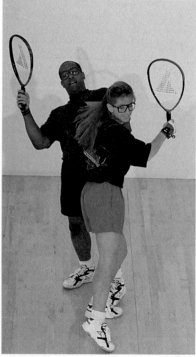

Figure 11.20 Two players colliding: dead-ball hinder.

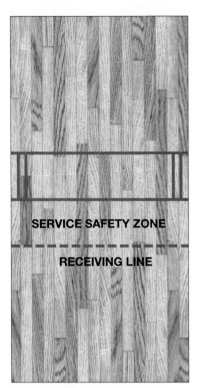

Figure 11.21 Five-foot safety zone.

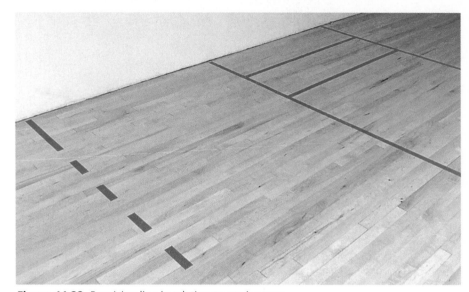

Figure 11.22 Receiving line in relation to service zone.

The etiquette of calling a dead-ball hinder rests initially with the player who creates the problem. That player's obligation is to state, "Do you want a hinder?" The response from the other player is either "Yes" or "No." If a hinder is identified by the offending player, the player restricted may say "Hinder please," and the opposing player has only the option of saying "Okay." In short, any request for a hinder is to be honored in an immediate affirmative manner. Hinders are to be requested immediately following the infraction so no question arises concerning whether a hinder should be called.

An avoidable hinder results in a point loss to the opponent if the opponent was receiving and committed the infraction, and a sideout if the infraction was made by the server. A dead-ball hinder requires a replay of the point. In a "friendly" game, avoidable hinders should seldom happen, as the idea of the game is to play for enjoyment and fitness. If a player does resort to committing avoidable hinders in such an environment, a judicial response is to not play that person again.

Miscellaneous Rules

The necessary rules interpretations include the use of the racquet. Often, beginners are not aware that the racquet must be held in one hand and remain in that hand throughout any specific rally. The racquet must also be attached to the wrist by the tether to reduce the possibility of injury. Another interpretation that is common knowledge, but that often is misunderstood, is that the ball must always be struck only by the racquet for a legal return. Other commonly misunderstood rules include the following:

1. The ball must be dry before being placed in play.

2. A server may not take a running stride to execute the serve.

3. A receiver of serve may not cross the receiving line and move into the safety zone until the served ball has crossed the short line, thus eliminating a potentially hazardous situation (see Figures 11.21 and 11.22).

4. A **crotch shot** strikes the crotch of the front wall and floor, ceiling or side wall simultaneously. During a serve, a crotch shot off the front wall is an out serve. A crotch shot serve that strikes off the floor and back wall, or the side wall and floor beyond the short line is in play.

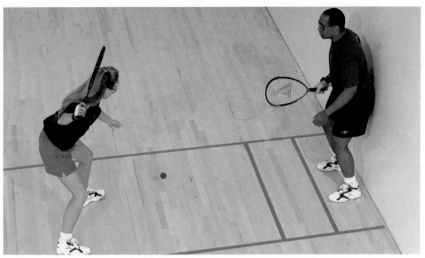

Figure 11.23 Doubles serving position.

During play, a crotch shot is always in play unless it hits the front wall.

5. Only the server is permitted to score after a winning rally.

Understanding the common rules of serving, hinders, and scoring allows the novice freedom to play the game early in skill development.

Beyond the Singles Game

The emphasis throughout this book has been on singles play. It is the safest form of racquetball, as there are just two players within an 800-square-foot area enclosed by four walls. Two additional games, however, are played with regularity in a four-wall court area. One is **doubles**, which is a competition between two-player teams. The other game is played with three players and is called **cut-throat**.

Doubles

Rules that relate to doubles are distinct in some ways, including serving order, player hitting order, position during serve, and hinder situations. The serve order follows a sequence of one partner serving consecutive points until a side-out occurs, and then the second partner

serving in a similar fashion until a second sideout takes place. The service order of the partners has one exception, and that fits only the first serving team. The first partner serves to the conclusion of serve, then the team exchanges with the receiving team. When the first serving team returns for the second round of serves, the first serving partner again begins serve, followed by the normal sequence of partner serve rotation.

The player hitting order, once the ball is placed in play by a serve, is the same as in the singles game, with team A hitting a serve, team B returning the serve, team A responding to return of serve, etc. Either player on a team may hit for that team in the rally.

During a serve, the serving team stands within the service zone as in singles play. One partner serves, and the other partner stands in the service box with his/her back to the side wall, or a foot-fault is called (see Figure 11.23).

If the partner in the doubles box is struck by the partner's serve, the serve is declared dead and the serve is executed again. Once the ball is in play, any ball that is hit by one partner and strikes the other partner is deemed a sideout or a handout if committed by the serving team, or a point for the serving team if committed by the receiving team. The receiving team must stand behind the receiving line to receive serve. Hinders are the same as in singles play, but the possibility for hinder calls is magnified by the presence of four players on the court at one time.

Cut-Throat

The cut-throat game is an unofficial racquetball game. One cut-throat game is a two-against-one setup, with the receiving team playing as a doubles team and the serving player competing against that team. Following each side-out, the doubles team membership changes, and the server becomes a part of a new doubles team. All play on the part of the doubles team as related to movement and position utilizes doubles rules, and all other play commences as in singles.

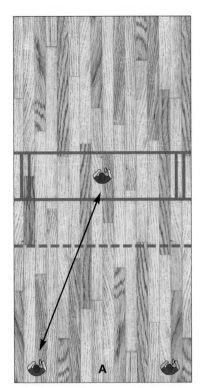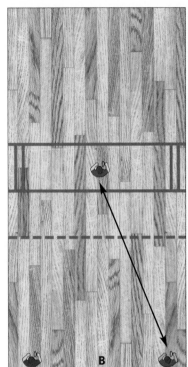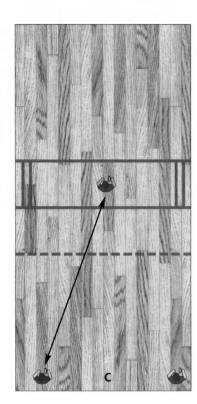

Figure 11.24 Serving rotation sequence.

The serving rotation follows a sequence of the server as the red player exchanging with the blue player, who is a receiver. When the next sideout occurs, the blue player, who has been the server, exchanges with the green player, who is the second receiver. The sequence follows an exchange of the green player (who is the server) on the next sideout with the red player, who has moved through the sequence as receiver. Then the process is repeated.

It should be noted that this type of exchange alternates the position of the receiver each time through the full serving sequence. If the blue receiver started from a right-side receiving position during the first sequence, that blue player would receive from the left side during the second sequence of return of serve (see Figure 11.24).

The second type of cut-throat game is a safer version and becomes a singles match with three players. One player is always sitting out a particular point by standing in a back-wall area while the other two players are playing. At the conclusion of each point, the non-competing player enters the game as a receiver of the serve, and the player who lost the point steps out. If the server loses the point, the former receiver becomes the server. If the receiver loses the point, the server remains as server, and play continues.

In both games of cut-throat, each player keeps an individual score, and the winner is the first player to gain 15 points. The game of cut-throat provides for a change-of-pace situation that permits three people to enjoy a game designed for two or four.

Three-Wall and One-Wall Racquetball

Racquetball can be played on other surfaces and configurations. Three-wall and one-wall games have developed in city parks and school playgrounds, and sometimes are found on college campuses where the weather is warm enough to provide for year-round play.

Racquetball played as a **three-wall** game follows the same rules as the four-wall game. Scoring, serving, ball in play, hinders, and all other general rules are the same. Exceptions to this are the result of the court structure itself, which does not have a back wall or a ceiling,

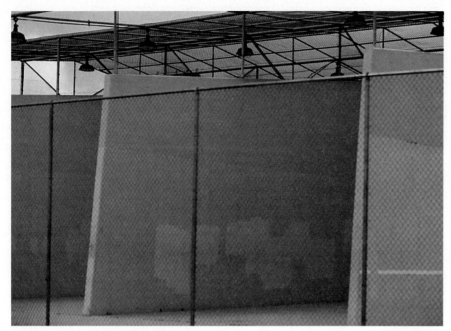

Figure 11.25 Three-wall racquetball court.

One-wall racquetball is also similar to the four-wall game. Obviously the major difference is that there are only two playing surfaces in the one-wall game; front wall and floor. The floor measures 20' wide and 34' long to the back edge of what is called the long line. The back edge of the short line is 16' from the front wall, and the service zone is all of the space between the short line and the front wall. With the exception of the court configuration, the game is played much as the four-wall game is played. Strategy is simplified to a power game since there are no rebound angles to play off side walls or ceiling.

and typically a side wall that does not extend completely to the long line (see Figure 11.25). These exceptions are presented below:

- A ball in play that lands outside the long line (where the back wall would normally be) is a point or sideout (or handout) depending on the situation.

- A served ball that lands outside the long line is a fault serve (long) just as in four-wall if the ball strikes the back wall on the fly.

- In the three-wall courts, where the side walls extend only partially to the long line, a serve or a ball in play hit wide of the side line is considered a wide ball and is a point or sideout (handout) depending on the situation.

- A ball in play or a served ball that is hit above the front wall (there is often a screen that catches the ball so players are not continually chasing the ball) is considered a point or sideout (handout).

- When the side wall does not extend fully to the long line, a hinder is called when a ball or player from an adjacent court crosses into a court with the ball in play.

Sportsmanship Ethic

Racquetball has a **sportsmanship ethic** that implies that the game is played for exercise and enjoyment. Coupled with that implication is the view that most matches are played without officiating, and it is imperative to call each point or shot fairly and without prejudice. It is doubly important to recognize that no point is worth winning if you or your opponent is injured.

The hinder is the best example of the application of sportsmanship, as many hinders have the potential for creating a circumstance that could result in injury. The hinder call allows for players to have a regard for the safety of their opponent and encourages a sportsmanship gesture because players call hinders on themselves and are expected to willingly accept a hinder call by their opponent.

The sportsmanship attitude extends to shaking hands following a match and being a "good loser" or "humble winner." The concept of sportsmanship is so much rhetoric in many other sports, but in racquetball, sportsmanship is required.

Points to Remember

→ When you warm up prior to playing, be sure to share the court in a side-by-side format.

→ A match consists of two 15-point games followed by a third game of 11 points if a tiebreaker is needed.

→ Winning a game requires only a one-point margin for victory.

→ A serve position originates from the service zone with a player's foot placed on or within the short and service lines.

→ Common fault serves include "short," "two-wall," and "long" serves resulting in a sideout if served in succession.

→ An out serve occurs in eight different situations, including the ball not initially striking the front wall, and is penalized by loss of serve.

→ A dead-ball hinder occurs as a result of unintentional action, and requires a replay of a rally.

→ An avoidable hinder occurs usually when one player intentionally or unintentionally creates an action that impedes the opponent, resulting in loss of the rally.

→ Racquetball can also be played as a doubles or cut-throat game.

→ Racquetball is played on indoor four-wall courts, and outdoor three-wall and one-wall courts.

→ Sportsmanship is required in racquetball for safety purposes, and because most matches are played on the honor system.

Self Testing Questions

Answers to Self Testing Questions are located on page 131.

1. Review this chapter and when you find a reference to a rule (e.g., see Rule 3.15 Avoidable Hinders), refer to the rules section of the book, and identify the specifics of the rules.

2. Analyze the type of games that can be played (i.e., singles, doubles, cut-throat, three-wall, and one-wall), and what differences exist between these games.

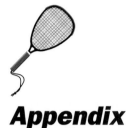

Appendix

2000 Official Rules of Racquetball

1—The Game

Rule 1.1 Types of Games

Racquetball is played by two or four players. When played by two, it is called singles and when played by four, doubles. A non-tournament variation of the game that is played by three players is called cutthroat.

Rule 1.2 Description

Racquetball is a competitive game in which a strung racquet is used to serve and return the ball.

Rule 1.3 Objective

The objective is to win each rally by serving or returning the ball so the opponent is unable to keep the ball in play. A rally is over when a player (or team in doubles) is unable to hit the ball before it touches the floor twice, is unable to return the ball in such a manner that it touches the front wall before it touches the floor, or when a hinder is called.

Rule 1.4 Points and Outs

Points are scored only by the serving side when it serves an irretrievable serve (an ace) or wins a rally. Losing the serve is called a sideout in singles. In doubles, when the first server loses the serve it is called a handout and when the second server loses the serve it is a sideout.

Rule 1.5 Match, Game, Tiebreaker

A match is won by the first side winning two games. The first two games of a match are played to 15 points. If each side wins one game, a tiebreaker game is played to 11 points.

2—Courts and Equipment

Rule 2.1 Court Specifications

The specifications for the standard four-wall racquetball court are:
(a) Dimensions. The dimensions shall be 20 feet wide, 40 feet long and 20 feet high, with a back wall at least 12 feet high. All surfaces shall be in play, with the exception of any gallery opening, surfaces designated as out-of-play for a valid reason (such as being of a very different material or not in alignment with the backwall), and designated court hinders.
(b) Markings. Racquetball courts shall be marked with lines 1½ inches wide as follows:
1. Short Line. The back edge of the short line is midway between, and parallel with, the front and back walls.
2. Service Line. The front edge of the service line is parallel with, and five feet in front of, the back edge of the short line.
3. Service Zone. The service zone is the 5' x 20' area

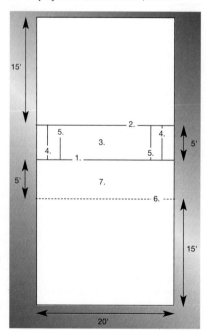

Reprinted with permission of The United States Racquetball Association, Colorado Springs, CO.

bounded by the bottom edges of the side walls and by the outer edges of the short line and the service line.

4. Service Boxes. The service boxes are located at each end of the service zone and are designated by lines parallel with the side walls [see 4.2(b)]. The edge of the line nearest to the center of the court shall be 18 inches from the nearest side wall.

5. Drive Serve Lines. The drive serve lines, which form the drive serve zone, are parallel with the side wall and are within the service zone. The edge of the line nearest to the center of the court shall be three feet from the nearest side wall.

6. Receiving Line. The receiving line is a broken line parallel to the short line. The back edge of the receiving line is five feet from the back edge of the short line. The receiving line begins with a line 21 inches long that extends from each side wall. These lines are connected by an alternate series of six-inch spaces and six-inch lines. This will result in a line composed of 17 six-inch spaces, 16 six-inch lines, and two 21-inch lines.

7. Safety Zone. The safety zone is the 5' x 20' area bounded by the bottom edges of the side walls and by the back edges of the short line and the receiving line. The zone is observed only during the serve. See Rules 3.10(i) and 3.11(a).

Rule 2.2 Ball Specifications

(a) The standard racquetball shall be 2¼ inches in diameter; weigh approximately 1.4 ounces, have a hardness of 55–60 inches durometer; and bounce 68–72 inches from a 100-inch drop at a temperature of 70–74 degrees Fahrenheit.

(b) Only a ball having the endorsement or approval of the USRA may be used in a USRA sanctioned tournament.

Rule 2.3 Ball Selection

(a) A ball shall be selected by the referee for use in each match. During the match the referee may, based on personal discretion or at the request of a player or team, replace the ball. Balls that are not round or which bounce erratically shall not be used.

(b) If possible, the referee and players should agree to an alternate ball, so that in the event of breakage, the second ball can be put into play immediately.

Rule 2.4 Racquet Specifications

(a) The racquet, including bumper guard and all solid parts of the handle, may not exceed 22 inches in length.

(b) The racquet frame may be any material judged to be safe.

(c) The racquet frame must include a cord that must be securely attached to the player's wrist.

(d) The string of the racquet must be gut, monofilament, nylon, graphite, plastic, metal, or a combination thereof, and must not mark or deface the ball.

(e) Using an illegal racquet will result in forfeiture of the game in progress or, if discovered between games, forfeiture of the preceding game.

Rule 2.5 Apparel

(a) All players must wear lensed eyewear that has been warranted by its manufacturer or distributor as 1.) designed for use in racquetball and 2.) meeting or exceeding either the full ASTM F803 standard or Canadian (CSA) impact standard. This rule applies to all persons, including those who wear corrective lenses. The eyewear must be unaltered and worn as designed at all times. A player who fails to wear proper eyewear will be assessed a technical foul and a timeout to obtain proper eyewear. A second infraction in the same match will result in immediate forfeiture of the match.

Certifications & Compliance. The USRA maintains a reference list of eyewear so warranted by their manufacturers, and provides that list to each sanctioned event (an eyewear list dated more than 90 days prior to the first day of the tournament will be deemed invalid for the purpose of determining compliance with this eyewear rule). In addition, the list is available online at the USRA.org website (indexed under "eyeguards"), and individual copies may be requested by calling the USRA National Office at 719/635-5396.

To be used in sanctioned competition, protective eyewear must:
- bear a permanent, physical stamp of the appropriate "ASTM-F803" citation on the frame itself, OR
- appear on the ASTM reference listing, OR
- bear the "Protective Eyewear Certification Council" [PECC] seal of approval for the ASTM standard, OR
- be certified in writing by the maker that it complies with the required ASTM standard (in this instance, the player must be able to provide written, adequate proof—on demand—at any sanctioned event, before such eyewear may be used).

(b) Clothing and Shoes. The clothing may be of any color; however, a player may be required to change wet, extremely loose fitting, or otherwise distracting garments. Insignias and writing on the clothing must be considered to be in good taste by the tournament director. Shoes must have soles which do not mark or damage the floor.

(c) Equipment Requirements During Warm-up. Proper eyeguards [see 2.5(a)] must be worn and wrist cords must be used during any on-court warm-up period. The referee should give a technical warning to any person who fails to comply and assess a technical foul if that player continues to not comply after receiving such a warning.

3—Play Regulations

Rule 3.1 Serve

In Open Division competition, the server will have one opportunity to put the ball into play [see section 5.0, for complete, one-serve modifications]. In all other divisions, the server will have two opportunities to put the ball into play.

The player or team winning the coin toss has the option to either serve or receive at the start of the first game. The second game will begin in reverse order of the first game. The player or team scoring the highest total of points in games 1 and 2 will have the option to serve or receive first at the start of the tiebreaker. In the event that both players or teams score an equal number of points in the first two games, another coin toss will take place and the winner of the toss will have the option to serve or receive.

Rule 3.2 Start

The server may not start the service motion until the referee has called the score or "second serve." The serve is started from any place within the service zone. (Certain drive serves are an exception. See Rule 3.6.) Neither the ball nor any part of either foot may extend beyond either line of the service zone when initiating the service motion. Stepping on, but not beyond, the lines is permitted. However, when completing the service motion, the server may step beyond the service (front) line provided that some part of both feet remain on or inside the line until the served ball passes the short line. The server may not step beyond the short line until the ball passes the short line. See Rule 3.9(a) and 3.10(i) for penalties for violations.

Rule 3.3 Manner

After taking a set position inside the service zone a player may begin the service motion—any continuous movement which results in the ball being served. Once the service motion begins, the ball must be bounced on the floor in the zone and be struck by the racquet before it bounces a second time. After being struck, the ball must hit the front wall first and on the rebound hit the floor beyond the back edge of the short line, either with or without touching one of the side walls.

Rule 3.4 Readiness

The service motion shall not begin until the referee has called the score or the second serve and the server has visually checked the receiver. The referee shall call the score as both server and receiver prepare to return to their respective positions, shortly after the previous rally has ended.

Rule 3.5 Delays

Except as noted in Rule 3.5(b), the referee may call a technical foul for delays exceeding 10 seconds.

(a) The 10 second rule applies to the server and receiver simultaneously. Collectively, they are allowed up to 10 seconds after the score is called to serve or be ready to receive. It is the server's responsibility to look and be certain the receiver is ready. If a receiver is not ready, they must signal by raising the racquet above the head or completely turning the back to the server. (These are the only two acceptable signals.)

(b) Serving while the receiving player/team is signaling "not ready" is a fault serve.

(c) After the score is called, if the server looks at the receiver and the receiver is not signalling "not ready", the server may then serve. If the receiver attempts to signal "not ready" after that point, the signal shall not be acknowledged and the serve becomes legal.

Rule 3.6 Drive Service Zones

The drive serve lines will be 3 feet from each side wall in the service zone. Viewed one at a time, the drive serve line divides the service area into a 3-foot and a 17-foot section that apply only to drive serves. The player may drive serve between the body and the side wall nearest to where the service motion began only if the player starts and remains outside of the 3-foot drive service zone. In the event that the service motion begins in one 3-foot drive service zone and continues into the other 3-foot drive serve zone, the player may not hit a drive serve at all.

(a) The drive serve zones are not observed for cross-court drive serves, the hard-Z, soft-Z, lob or half-lob serves.

(b) The racquet may not break the plane of the 17-foot zone while making contact with the ball.

(c) The drive serve line is not part of the 17-foot zone. Dropping the ball on the line or standing on the line while serving to the same side is an infraction.

Rule 3.7 Defective Serves

Defective serves are of three types resulting in penalties as follows:

(a) Dead-Ball Serve. A dead-ball serve results in no penalty and the server is given another serve (without cancelling a prior fault serve).

(b) Fault Serve. Two fault serves result in an out (either a sideout or a handout).

(c) Out Serve. An out serve results in an out (either a sideout or a handout).

Rule 3.8 Dead-Ball Serves

Dead-ball serves do not cancel any previous fault serve. The following are dead-ball serves:

(a) Court Hinders. A serve that takes an irregular bounce because it hit a wet spot or an irregular surface on the court is a dead-ball serve. Also, any serve that hits any surface designated by local rules as an obstruction rather than being out-of-play.

(b) Broken Ball. If the ball is determined to have broken on the serve, a new ball shall be substituted and the serve shall be replayed, not canceling any prior fault serve.

Rule 3.9 Fault Serves

The following serves are faults and any two in succession result in an out:

(a) Foot Faults. A foot fault results when:
1. The server does not begin the service motion with both feet in the service zone.
2. The server steps completely over the service line (no part of the foot on or inside the service zone) before the served ball crosses the short line.

(b) Short Service. A short serve is any served ball that first hits the front wall and, on the rebound, hits the floor on or in front of the short line either with or without touching a side wall.

(c) Three Wall Serve. A three-wall serve is any served ball that first hits the front wall and, on the rebound, strikes both side walls before touching the floor.

(d) Ceiling Serve. A ceiling serve is any served ball that first hits the front wall and then touches the ceiling (with or without touching a side wall).

(e) Long Serve. A long serve is a served ball that first hits the front wall and rebounds to the back wall before touching the floor (with or without touching a side wall).

(f) Bouncing Ball Outside Service Zone. Bouncing the ball outside the service zone as a part of the service motion is a fault serve.

(g) Illegal Drive Serve. A drive serve in which the player fails to observe the 17-foot drive service zone outlined in Rule 3.6.

(h) Screen Serve. A served ball that first hits the front wall and on the rebound passes so closely to the server, or server's partner in doubles, that it prevents the receiver from having a clear view of the ball. (The receiver is obligated to take up good court position, near center court, to obtain that view.)

(i) In open division play, if a serve is called a screen, the server will be allowed one more opportunity to hit a legal serve. Two consecutive screen serves results in an out.

Rule 3.10 Out Serves

Any of the following results in an out:

(a) Two Consecutive Fault Serves [see Rule 3.9], *or a single fault serve in open division play [see exceptions: 5.0].*

(b) Missed Serve Attempt. Any attempt to strike the ball that results in a total miss or in the ball touching any part of the server's body. Also, allowing the ball to bounce more than once during the service motion.

(c) Touched Serve. Any served ball that on the rebound from the front wall touches the server or server's racquet before touching the floor, or any ball intentionally stopped or caught by the server or server's partner.

(d) Fake or Balk Serve. Any movement of the racquet toward the ball during the serve which is non-continuous and done for the purpose of deceiving the receiver. If a balk serve occurs, but the referee believes that no deceit was involved, the option of declaring "no serve" and having the serve replayed without penalty can be exercised.

(e) Illegal Hit. An illegal hit includes contacting the ball twice, carrying the ball, or hitting the ball with the handle of the racquet or part of the body or uniform.

(f) Non-Front Wall Serve. Any served ball that does not strike the front wall first.

(g) Crotch Serve. Any served ball that hits the crotch of the front wall and floor, front wall and side wall, or front wall and ceiling is an out serve (because it did not hit the front wall first). A serve into the crotch of the back wall and floor is a good serve and in play. A served ball that hits the crotch of the side wall and floor beyond the short line is in play.

(h) Out-of-Court Serve. An out-of-court serve is any served ball that first hits the front wall and, before striking the floor, either goes out of the court or hits a surface above the normal playing area of the court that has been declared as out-of-play for a valid reason [See Rule 2.1(a)].

(i) Safety Zone Violation. If the server, or doubles partner, enters into the safety zone before the served ball passes the short line, it shall result in the loss of serve.

Rule 3.11 Return of Serve

(a) Receiving Position
1. The receiver may not enter the safety zone until the ball bounces or crosses the receiving line.
2. On the fly return attempt, the receiver may not strike the ball until the ball breaks the plane of the receiving line. However, the receiver's follow-through may carry the receiver or the racquet past the receiving line.
3. Neither the receiver nor the racquet may break the plane of the short line, except if the ball is struck after rebounding off the back wall.
4. Any violation by the receiver results in a point for the server.

(b) Defective Serve. A player on the receiving side may not intentionally catch or touch a served ball (such as an apparently long or short serve) until the referee has made a call or the ball has touched the floor for a second time. Violation results in a point.

(c) Legal Return. After a legal serve, a player receiving the serve must strike the ball on the fly or after the first bounce, and before the ball touches the floor the second time; and return the ball to the front wall, either directly or after touching one or both side walls, the back wall or the ceiling, or any combination of those surfaces. A returned ball must touch the front wall before touching the floor.

(d) Failure to Return. The failure to return a serve results in a point for the server.

(e) Other Provisions. Except as noted in this rule (3.11), the return of serve is subject to all provisions of Rules 3.13 through 3.15.

Rule 3.12 Changes of Serve

(a) Outs. A server is entitled to continue serving until one of the following occurs:

1. Out Serve. See Rule 3.10.
2. Two Consecutive Fault Serves [see Rule 3.9], *or a single fault serve in open division play [see exceptions: 5.0].*
3. Failure to Return Ball. Player or team fails to keep the ball in play as required by Rule 3.11 (c).
4. Avoidable Hinder. Player or team commits an avoidable hinder which results in an out. See Rule 3.15.

(b) Sideout. Retiring the server in singles is called a sideout.

(c) Effect of Sideout. When the server (or serving team) receives a sideout, the server becomes the receiver and the receiver becomes the server.

Rule 3.13 Rallies

All of the play which occurs after the successful return of serve is called the rally. Play shall be conducted according to the following rules:

(a) Legal Hits. Only the head of the racquet may be used at any time to return the ball. The racquet may be held in one or both hands. Switching hands to hit a ball, touching the ball with any part of the body or uniform, or removing the wrist safety cord during a rally results in a loss of the rally.

(b) One Touch. The player or team trying to return the ball may touch or strike the ball only once or else the rally is lost. The ball may not be carried. (A carried ball is one which rests on the racquet long enough that the effect is more of a sling or throw than a hit.)

(c) Failure to Return. Any of the following constitutes a failure to make a legal return during a rally:

1. The ball bounces on the floor more than once before being hit.
2. The ball does not reach the front wall on the fly.
3. The ball is hit such that it goes into the gallery or wall opening or else hits a surface above the normal playing area of the court that has been declared as out-of-play. See Rule 2.1(a).
4. A ball which obviously does not have the velocity or direction to hit the front wall strikes another player.
5. A ball struck by one player on a team hits that player or that player's partner.
6. Committing an avoidable hinder. See Rule 3.15.
7. Switching hands during a rally.
8. Failure to use a racquet wrist safety cord.
9. Touching the ball with the body or uniform.
10. Carrying or slinging the ball with the racquet.

(d) Effect of Failure to Return. Violations of Rules 3.13 (a) through (c) result in a loss of rally. If the serving player or team loses the rally, it is an out. If the receiver loses the rally, it results in a point for the server.

(e) Return Attempts. The ball remains in play until it touches the floor a second time, regardless of how many walls it makes contact with—including the front wall. If a player swings at the ball and misses it, the player may continue to attempt to return the ball until it touches the floor for the second time.

(f) Broken Ball. If there is any suspicion that a ball has broken during a rally, play shall continue until the end of the rally. The referee or any player may request the ball be examined. If the referee decides the ball is broken the ball will be replaced and the rally replayed. The server resumes play at first serve. The only proper way to check for a broken ball is to squeeze it by hand. (Checking the ball by striking it with a racquet will not be considered a valid check and shall work to the disadvantage of the player or team which struck the ball after the rally.)

(g) Play Stoppage

1. If a foreign object enters the court, or any other outside interference occurs, the referee shall stop the play immediately and declare a dead-ball hinder.
2. If a player loses any apparel, equipment, or other article, the referee shall stop play immediately and declare an avoidable hinder or dead-ball hinder as described in Rule 3.15 (i).

(h) Replays. Whenever a rally is replayed for any reason, the server resumes play at first serve. A previous fault serve is not considered.

Rule 3.14 Dead-Ball Hinders

A rally is replayed without penalty and the server resumes play at first serve whenever a dead-ball hinder occurs. Also, see Rule 3.15 which describes conditions under which a hinder might be declared avoidable and result in loss of the rally.

(a) Situations

1. Court Hinders. The referee should stop play immediately whenever the ball hits any part of the court that was designated in advance as a court hinder (such as a vent grate). The referee should also stop play (i) when the ball takes an irregular bounce as a result of contacting a rough surface (such as court light or vent) or after striking a wet spot on the floor or wall and (ii) when, in the referee's opinion, the irregular bounce affected the rally.

2. Ball Hits Opponent. When an opponent is hit by a return shot in flight, it is a dead-ball hinder. If the opponent is struck by a ball which obviously did not have the velocity or direction to reach the front wall, it is not a hinder, and the player who hit the ball will lose the rally. A player who has been hit by the ball can stop play and make the call though the call must be made immediately and acknowledged by the referee. Note this interference may, under certain conditions, be declared an avoidable hinder. See Rule 3.15.

3. Body Contact. If body contact occurs which the referee believes was sufficient to stop the rally, either for the purpose of preventing injury by further contact or because the contact prevented a player from being able to make a reasonable return, the referee shall call a hinder. Incidental body contact in which the offensive player clearly will have the advantage should not be called a hinder, unless the offensive player obviously stops play. Contact with the racquet on the follow-through normally is not considered a hinder.

4. Screen Ball. Any ball rebounding from the front wall so close to the body of the defensive player that it prevents the offensive player from having a clear view of the ball. (The referee should be careful not to make the screen call so quickly that it takes away a good offensive opportunity.) A ball that passes between the legs of a player who has just returned the ball is not automatically a screen. It depends on whether the other player is impaired as a result. Generally, the call should work to the advantage of the offensive player.

5. Backswing Hinder. Any body or racquet contact, on the backswing or on the way to or just prior to returning the ball, which impairs the hitter's ability to take a reasonable swing. This call can be made by the player attempting the return, though the call must be made immediately and is subject to the referee's approval. Note the interference may be considered an avoidable hinder. See Rule 3.15.

6. Safety Holdup. Any player about to execute a return who believes that striking the opponent with the ball or racquet is likely, may immediately stop play and request a dead-ball hinder. This call must be made immediately and is subject to acceptance and approval of the referee. (The referee will grant a dead-ball hinder if it is believed the holdup was reasonable and the player would have been able to return the shot. The referee may also call an avoidable hinder if warranted.)

7. Other Interference. Any other unintentional interference which prevents an opponent from having a fair chance to see or return the ball. Example: When a ball from another court enters the court during a rally or when a referee's call on an adjacent court obviously distracts a player.

(b) Effect of Hinders. The referee's call of hinder stops play and voids any situation which follows, such as the ball hitting the player. The only hinders that may be called by a player are described in rules (2), (5), and (6) above, and all of these are subject to the approval of the referee. A dead-ball hinder stops play and the rally is replayed. The server receives two serves.

(c) Responsibility. While making an attempt to return the ball, a player is entitled to a fair chance to see and return the ball. It is the responsibility of the side that has just hit the ball to move so the receiving side may go straight to the ball and have an unobstructed view of and swing at the ball. However, the receiver is responsible for making a reasonable effort to move towards the ball and must have a reasonable chance to return the ball for any type of hinder to be called.

Rule 3.15 Avoidable Hinders

An avoidable hinder results in the loss of the rally. An avoidable hinder does not necessarily have to be an intentional act. Dead-ball hinders are described in Rule 3.14. Any of the following results in an avoidable hinder:

(a) Failure to Move. A player does not move sufficiently to allow an opponent a shot straight to the front wall as well as a cross-court shot which is a shot directly to the front wall at an angle that would cause the ball to rebound directly to the rear corner farthest from the player hitting the ball. Also when a player moves in such a direction that it prevents an opponent from taking either of these shots.

(b) Stroke Interference. This occurs when a player moves, or fails to move, so that the opponent returning the ball does not have a free, unimpeded swing. This includes unintentionally moving in a direction which prevents the opponent from making an open, offensive shot.

(c) Blocking. Moves into a position which blocks the opponent from getting to, or returning, the ball; or in doubles, a player moves in front of an opponent as the player's partner is returning the ball.

(d) Moving into the Ball. Moves in the way and is struck by the ball just played by the opponent.

(e) Pushing. Deliberately pushes or shoves opponent during a rally.

(f) Intentional Distractions. Deliberate shouting, stamping of feet, waving of racquet, or any other manner of disrupting one's opponent.

(g) View Obstruction. A player moves across an opponent's line of vision just before the opponent strikes the ball.

(h) Wetting the Ball. The players, particularly the server, should ensure that the ball is dry prior to the serve. Any wet ball that is not corrected prior to the serve shall result in an avoidable hinder against the server.

(i) Apparel or Equipment Loss. If a player loses any apparel, equipment, or other article, play shall be immediately stopped and that player shall be called for an avoidable hinder, unless the player has just hit a shot that could not be retrieved. If the loss of equipment is caused by a player's opponent, then a dead-ball hinder should be called. If the opponent's action is judged to have been avoidable, then the opponent should be called for an avoidable hinder.

Rule 3.16 Timeouts

(a) Rest Periods. Each player or team is entitled to three 30-second timeouts in games to 15 and two 30-second timeouts in games to 11. Timeouts may not be called by either side after service motion has begun. Calling for a timeout when none remain or after service motion has begun, or taking more than 30 seconds in a timeout, will result in the assessment of a technical foul for delay of game.

(b) Injury. If a player is injured during the course of a match as a result of contact, such as with the ball, racquet, wall or floor an injury timeout will be awarded. While a player may call more than one timeout for the same injury or for additional injuries which occur during the match, a player is not allowed more than a total of 15 minutes of rest for injury during the entire match. If the injured player is not able to resume play after total rest of 15 minutes, the match shall be awarded to the opponent.

1. Should any external bleeding occur, the referee must halt play as soon as the rally is over, charge an injury timeout to the person who is bleeding, and not allow the match to continue until the bleeding has stopped.
2. Muscle cramps and pulls, fatigue, and other ailments that are not caused by direct contact on the court will not be considered an injury. Injury time is also not allowed for pre-existing conditions.

(c) Equipment Timeouts. Players are expected to keep all clothing and equipment in good, playable condition and are expected to use regular timeouts and time between games for adjustment and replacement of equipment. If a player or team is out of timeouts and the referee determines that an equipment change or adjustment is necessary for fair and safe continuation of the match, the referee may grant an equipment timeout not to exceed 2 minutes. The referee may allow additional time under unusual circumstances.

(d) Between Games. The rest period between the first two games of a match is 2 minutes. If a tiebreaker is necessary, the rest period between the second and third game is 5 minutes.

(e) Postponed Games. Any games postponed by referees shall be resumed with the same score as when postponed.

Rule 3.17 Technical Fouls and Warnings

(a) Technical Fouls. The referee is empowered to deduct one point from a player's or team's score when, in the referee's sole judgment, the player is being overtly and deliberately abusive. If the player or team against whom the technical foul was assessed does not resume play immediately, the referee is empowered to forfeit the match in favor of the opponent. Some examples of actions which can result in technical fouls are:

1. Profanity.
2. Excessive arguing.
3. Threat of any nature to opponent or referee.
4. Excessive or hard striking of the ball between rallies.
5. Slamming of the racquet against walls or floor, slamming the door, or any action which might result in damage to the court or injury to other players.
6. Delay of game. Examples include (i) taking too much time to dry the court, (ii) excessive questioning of the referee about the rules, (iii) exceeding the time allotted for timeouts or between games, (iv) calling a timeout when none remain, or after the service motion begins, or (v) taking more than ten seconds to serve or be ready to receive serve.
7. Intentional front line foot fault to negate a bad lob serve.
8. Anything the referee considers to be unsportsmanlike behavior.
9. Failure to wear lensed eyewear designed for racquet sports [See Rule 2.5(a)] is an automatic technical foul on the first infraction, plus a mandatory timeout (to acquire the proper eyewear) will be charged against the offending player. A second infraction by that player during the match will result in automatic forfeiture of the match.

(b) Technical Warnings. If a player's behavior is not so severe as to warrant a technical foul, a technical warning may be issued without the deduction of a point.

(c) Effect of Technical Foul or Warning. If a referee issues a technical foul, one point shall be removed from the offender's score. No point will be deducted if a referee issues a technical warning. In either case, a technical foul or warning should be accompanied by a brief explanation. Issuing a technical foul or warning has no effect on who will be serving when play resumes. If a technical foul occurs when the offender has no points or between games, the result will be that the offender's score becomes minus one (-1).

Rule Modifications

The following sections (4.0 through 11.0) detail the additional or modified rules that apply to variations of the singles game described in Sections 1 through 3.

4.0—Doubles

The USRA's rules for singles also apply in doubles with the following additions and modifications:

Rule 4.1 Doubles Team

(a) A doubles team shall consist of two players who meet either the age requirements or player classification requirements to participate in a particular division of play. A team with different skill levels must play in the division of the player with the higher level of ability. When playing in an adult age division, the team must play in the division of the younger player. When playing in a junior age division, the team must play in the division of the older player.

(b) A change in playing partners may be made so long as the first match of the posted team has not begun. For this purpose only, the match will be considered started once the teams have been called to the court. The team must notify the tournament director of the change prior to the beginning of the match.

Rule 4.2 Serve in Doubles

(a) Order of Serve. Each team shall inform the referee the order of service which shall be followed throughout that game. The order of serve may be changed between games, provided that the referee has been verbally notified before the first serve of the new game. At the beginning of each game, when the first server of the first team is out, the team is out. Therefore, both players on each team shall serve until the team receives a handout and a sideout.

(b) Partner's Position. On each serve, the server's partner shall stand erect with back to the side wall and with both feet on the floor within the service box from the moment the server begins the service motion until the served ball passes the short line. Violations are called foot faults. However, if the server's partner enters the safety zone before the ball passes the short line, the server loses service.

(c) Changes of Serve. In doubles, the side is retired when both partners have lost service, except that the team which serves first at the beginning of each game loses the serve when the first server is retired.

Rule 4.3 Fault Serve in Doubles

(a) The server's partner is not in the service box with both feet on the floor and back to the side wall from the time the server begins the service motion until the ball passes the short line.

(b) A served ball that hits the doubles partner while in the doubles box results in a fault serve.

(c) In open division play, if a serve hits the non-serving partner while standing in the box, the server will be allowed one more opportunity to hit a legal serve. Hitting the non-serving partner twice results in an out.

(d) In open division play, consecutive faults—either (i) a screen serve followed by hitting the non-serving partner or (ii) hitting the non-serving partner followed by a screen serve—results in an out.

Rule 4.4 Out Serve in Doubles

(a) Out-of-Order Service. In doubles, when either partner serves out of order, the points scored by that server will be subtracted and an out serve will be called: if the second server serves out of order, the out serve will be applied to the first server and the second server will resume serving. If the player designated as the first server serves out of order, a sideout will be called. The referee should call "no serve" as soon as an out-of-order serve occurs. If no points are scored while the team is out of order, only the out penalty will have to assessed. However, if points are scored before the out of order condition is noticed and the referee cannot recall the number, the referee may enlist the aid of the line judges (but not the crowd) to recall the number of points to be deducted.

(b) Ball Hits Partner. A served ball that hits the doubles partner while outside the doubles box results in loss of serve.

Rule 4.5 Return in Doubles

(a) The rally is lost if one player hits that same player's partner with an attempted return.

(b) If one player swings at the ball and misses it, both partners may make further attempts to return the ball until it touches the floor the second time. Both partners on a side are entitled to return the ball.

5.0—One Serve

The USRA's standard rules governing racquetball play will be followed, but only one serve is allowed. Therefore, any fault serve is an out serve, with a few exceptions [noted separately below, and within the text rules cited].

See Rule 3.9 Fault Serves
[Screens]
(a) In open division play, if a serve is called a screen, the server will be allowed one more opportunity to hit a legal serve. Two consecutive screen serves results in an out.

See Rule 4.3 Fault Serves in Doubles
[Serve hits partner]
(b) In open division play, if a serve hits the non-serving partner while standing in the box, the server will be allowed one more opportunity to hit a legal serve. Hitting the non-serving partner twice, results in an out.

[Consecutive faults]
(c) In open division play, consecutive faults—either (i) a screen serve followed by hitting the non-serving partner or (ii) hitting the non-serving partner followed by a screen serve—results in an out.

6.0—Multi-Bounce

In general, the USRA's standard rules governing racquetball play will be followed except for the modifications which follow.

Rule 6.1 Basic Return Rule

In general, the ball remains in play as long as it is bouncing. However, the player may swing only once at the ball and the ball is considered dead at the point it stops bouncing and begins to roll. Also, anytime the ball rebounds off the back wall, it must be struck before it crosses the short line on the way to the front wall, except as explained in Rule 6.2.

Rule 6.2 Blast Rule

If the ball caroms from the front wall to the back wall on the fly, the player may hit the ball from any place on the court—including past the short line—so long as the ball is still bouncing.

Rule 6.3 Front Wall Lines

Two parallel lines (tape may be used) should be placed across the front wall such that the bottom edge of one line is 3 feet above the floor and the bottom edge of the other line is 1 foot above the floor. During the rally any ball that hits the front wall (i) below the 3-foot line and (ii) either on or above the 1-foot line must be returned before it bounces a third time. However, if the ball hits below the 1-foot line, it must be returned before it bounces twice. If the ball hits on or above the 3-foot line, the ball must be returned as described in the basic return rule.

Rule 6.4 Games and Matches

All games are played to 11 points and the first side to win two games, wins the match.

7.0—One-Wall and Three-Wall Play

In general the USRA's standard rules governing racquetball play will be followed except the modifications which follow.

Rule 7.1 One-Wall

There are two playing surfaces—the front wall and the floor. The wall is 20 feet wide and 16 feet high. The floor is 20 feet wide and 34 feet to the back edge of the long line. To permit movement by players, there should be a minimum of three feet (six feet is recommended) beyond the long line and six feet outside each side line.

(a) Short Line. The back edge of the short line is 16 feet from the wall.

(b) Service Markers. Lines at least six inches long which are parallel with, and midway between the long and short lines. The extension of the service markers form the imaginary boundary of the service line.

(c) Service Zone. The entire floor area inside and including the short line, side lines and service line.

(d) Receiving Zone. The entire floor area in back of the short line including the side lines and the long line.

Rule 7.2 Three Wall

(a) Short Side Wall. The front wall is 20 feet wide and 20 feet high. The side walls are 20 feet long and 20 feet high, with the side walls tapering to 12 feet high. The floor length and court markings are the same as a four wall court.

(b) Long Side Wall. The court is 20 feet wide, 20 feet high and 40 feet long. The side walls may taper from 20 feet high at the front wall down to 12 feet high at the end of the court. All court markings are the same as a four wall court.

(c) Three wall service. A serve that goes beyond the side walls on the fly is an out. A serve that goes beyond the long line on a fly but within the side walls, is a fault.

8.0—Wheelchair

In general, the USRA's standard rules governing racquetball play will be followed, except for the modifications which follow.

Rule 8.1 Modifications

(a) Where USRA rules refer to server, person, body, or other similar variations, for wheelchair play such reference shall include all parts of the wheelchair in addition to the person sitting on it.

(b) Where the rules refer to feet, standing or other similar descriptions, for wheelchair play it means only where the rear wheels actually touch the floor.

(c) Where the rules mention body contact, for wheelchair play it shall mean any part of the wheelchair in addition to the player.

(d) Where the rules refer to double bounce or after the first bounce, it shall mean three bounces. All variations of the same phrases shall be revised accordingly.

Rule 8.2 Divisions

(a) Novice Division. The novice division is for the beginning player who is just learning to play.

(b) Intermediate Division. The Intermediate Division is for the player who has played tournaments before and has a skill level to be competitive in the division.

(c) Open Division. The Open Division is the highest level of play and is for the advanced player.

(d) Multi-Bounce Division. The Multi-Bounce Division is for the individuals (men or women) whose mobility is such that wheelchair racquetball would be impossible if not for the Multi-Bounce Division.

(e) Junior Division. The junior divisions are for players who are under the age of 19. The tournament director will determine if the divisions will be played as two bounce or multi-bounce. Age divisions are: 8–11, 12–15, and 16–18.

Rule 8.3 Rules

(a) Two Bounce Rule. Two bounces are used in wheelchair racquetball in all divisions except the Multi-Bounce Division. The ball may hit the floor twice before being returned.

(b) Out-of-Chair Rule. The player can neither intentionally jump out of the chair to hit a ball nor stand up in the chair to serve the ball. If the referee determines that the chair was left intentionally it will result in loss of the rally for the offender. If a player unintentionally leaves the chair, no penalty will be assessed. Repeat offenders will be warned by the referee.

(c) Equipment Standards. To protect playing surfaces, the tournament officials will not allow a person to participate with black tires or anything which will mark or damage the court.

(d) Start. The serve may be started from any place within the service zone. Although the front casters may extend beyond the lines of the service zone, at no time shall the rear wheels cross either the service or short line before the served ball crosses the short line. Penalties for violation are the same as those for the standard game.

(e) Maintenance Delay. A maintenance delay is a delay in the progress of a match due to a malfunction of a wheelchair, prosthesis, or assistive device. Such delay must be requested by the player, granted by the referee during the match, and shall not exceed 5 minutes. Only two such delays may be granted for each player for each match. After using both maintenance delays, the player has the following options: (i) continue play with the defective equipment, (ii) immediately substitute replacement equipment, or (iii) postpone the game, with the approval of the referee and opponent.

Rule 8.4 Multi-Bounce Rules

(a) The ball may bounce as many times as the receiver wants though the player may swing only once to return the ball to the front wall.

(b) The ball must be hit before it crosses the short line on its way back to the front wall.

(c) The receiver cannot cross the short line after the ball contacts the back wall.

9.0—Visually Impaired

In general, the USRA's standard rules governing racquetball play will be followed except for the modifications which follow.

Rule 9.1 Eligibility

A player's visual acuity must not be better than 20/200 with the best practical eye correction or else the player's field of vision must not be better than 20 degrees. The three classifications of blindness are B1 (totally blind to light perception), B2 (able to see hand movement up to 20/600 corrected), and B3 (from 20/600 to 20/200 corrected).

Rule 9.2 Return of Serve and Rallies

On the return of serve and on every return thereafter, the player may make multiple attempts to strike the ball until (i) the ball has been touched, (ii) the ball has stopped bouncing, or (iii) the ball has passed the short line after touching the back wall. The only exception is described in Rule 9.3

Rule 9.3 Blast Rule

If the ball (other than on the serve) caroms from the front wall to the back wall on the fly, the player may retrieve the ball from any place on the court—including in front of the short line—so long as the ball has not been touched and is still bouncing.

Rule 9.4 Hinders

A dead-ball hinder will result in the rally being replayed without penalty unless the hinder was intentional. If a hinder is clearly intentional an avoidable hinder should be called and the rally awarded to the non-offending player or team.

10.0—Deaf

In general, the USRA's standard rules governing racquetball play will be followed except for the modifications which follow.

Rule 10.1 Eligibility

An athlete shall have a hearing loss of 55 db or more in the better ear to be eligible for any tournament for deaf athletes.

11.0—Men's Professional [International Racquetball Tour/IRT]

In general, competition on the International Racquetball Tour [IRT] will follow the standard rules governing racquetball established by the USRA, except for the modifications which follow. Modifications for both professional tours are consistent, with one exception as noted in Rule 11.4.

Rule 11.1 Game, Match

All games are played to 11 points, and are won by the player who scores to that level, with a 2-Point lead. If necessary the game will continue beyond 11 points, until such time as one player has a 2-point lead. Matches are played the best three out of a possible five games to 11.

Rule 11.2 Appeals

The referee's call is final. There are no line judges, and no appeals may be made.

Rule 11.3 Serve

Players are allowed only one serve to put the ball into play.

Rule 11.4 Screen Serve

In IRT matches, screen serves are replayed. In WIRT matches, two consecutive screen serves will result in a side-out.

Rule 11.5 Court Hinders

No court hinders are allowed or called.

Rule 11.6 Out-of-Court Ball

Any ball leaving the court results in a loss of rally.

Rule 11.7 Ball

All matches are played with the Pro Penn ball. The first, third, and fifth (if necessary) games of the match are started with a new ball.

Rule 11.8 Timeouts

(a) Per Game. Each player is entitled to one 1-minute timeout per game.
(b) Between Points. The player has 15 seconds from the end of the previous rally to put the ball in play.
(c) Between Games. The rest period between all games is 2 minutes, including a fifth game tiebreaker.
(d) Equipment Timeouts. A player does not have to use regular timeouts to correct or adjust equipment, provided that the need for the change or adjustment is acknowledged by the referee as being necessary for fair and safe continuation of the match.
(e) Injury Timeout. Consists of two 7½ minute timeouts within a match. Once an injury timeout is taken, the full 7½ minutes must be used, or it is forfeited.

12.0—Women's Professional [Ladies Professional Racquetball Association/LPRA]

In general, competition in the Ladies Professional Racquetball Association [LPRA] will follow the standard rules governing racquetball established by the USRA, except for the modifications which follow.

Rule 12.1 Game, Match

All games are played to 11 points, and are won by the player who scores to that level, with a 2-point lead. If necessary, the game will continue beyond 11 points, until such time as one player has a 2-point lead. Matches are played the best three out of a possible five games to 11.

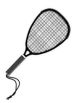

Answer Key to Self Testing Questions

Chapter 1
1. c
2. b
3. d
4. d
5. d
6. d
7. c
8. Refer to the list on pages 6–7

Chapter 2
1. a
2. b
3. d
4. b
5. b
6. refer to upper body stretch area on pp. 17–18
7. Refer to lower body stretch area on pp. 18–19
8. a

Chapter 3
1. a
2. b
3. d
4. b
5. a
6. b
7. d
8. a

Chapter 4
1. a
2. b
3. a
4. b
5. c
6. b
7. a
8. c

Chapter 5
1. b
2. d
3. d
4. d
5. c
6. F
7. F
8. T
9. T
10. F
11. T
12. F
13. T
14. F

Chapter 6
1. c
2. b
3. d
4. T
5. T
6. T

7. F
8. T
9. F
10. T
11. T
12. F
13. F

Chapter 7
1. d
2. a
3. d
4. T
5. F
6. F
7. T

Chapter 8
1. a
2. d
3. T
4. T
5. F
6. F

Chapter 9
1. d
2. d
3. T
4. T
5. F

Glossary of Terms

Ace: A legal serve that the receiver of the serve totally missed.

Alley: The lane along the side walls that is a target for down-the-line passing shots.

Around-the-Wall Ball: A defensive shot that hits three walls before touching the floor.

Avoidable Hinder: Interference with the opponent's opportunity to play a shot fairly, including failure to move, stroke interference, blocking, moving into the ball, pushing, intentional distractions, obstruction of view, and wetting of the ball.

Back Court: That section of the court nearest the back wall and described as the last third of the court.

Backhand: A stroke hit from the non-racquet side of the body.

Backswing: The preparation phase of the basic swing.

Back Wall: The rear wall, usually the entrance to the court area.

Ceiling Shot: A ball that strikes ceiling–front wall in sequence.

Center Court: The area immediately behind the short line and equal distance from the side walls.

Closed Face: Position of the racquet face on the ball when hitting the ball downward (usually turned away from the ceiling).

Continental Grip: The grip positioned halfway between the Eastern Forehand and the backhand grip.

Corner Kill Shot: A kill shot that strikes the front wall–side wall and rebounds into the direction of mid-court.

Cross-Court Shot: A two-wall passing shot executed when the opponent is either on the same side as you or is in an "up" position. The ball hits front wall and then side wall.

Crotch Shot: A ball striking two playing surfaces simultaneously (such as wall and floor).

Cut-throat: A three-player racquetball game designed with the server playing against the other two players.

Dead-Ball Hinder: An unintentional interference with the opponent's opportunity to play a shot fairly, including: court hinders, ball hitting an opponent, body contact, screen ball, backswing hinder, and a safety holdup.

Defensive Shots: Shots that prevent the opponent from holding an offensive court position.

Dehydration: Condition brought on by loss of body fluids.

Doubles: A four-player racquetball game played between teams of two players.

Down-the-line Passing Shot: A shot that carries along a side wall 1 to 2 feet from the wall and below the opponent's waist. This also is called down-the-wall and it is designed to pass an opponent who is in an "up" position.

Drive: A powerfully hit shot that follows a straight path off the front wall.

Drive Serve: A powerfully hit serve that follows a straight path off the front wall.

Drive Serve Zone: The zone defined by two lines 3 feet from each side wall in the service box that divides the service zone into two 17-foot service zones for drive serves. The zone is associated with the special rule regarding drive serves.

Drop Shot: A touch shot that is hit with deception and little force.

Eastern Backhand Grip: The conventional backhand grip that is assumed by rotating the racquet a quarter turn to the racquet side of the body from the Eastern Forehand grip.

Eastern Forehand Grip: The conventional racquetball grip best described as a "shake hands" position.

Fault: A serve that touches the floor before passing the short line, or one in which the ball strikes the front wall and the ceiling, the back wall, or two side walls before hitting the floor. These serves are illegal and must be replayed. Two faults result in a sideout.

Flexibility: Ease and range of movement.

Follow-through: Arm movement after hitting the ball.

Foot Fault: An illegal serve identified by the server's foot touching the outside of the service area, or in doubles when the server's partner is not positioned in the service box during the serve.

Forehand: A stroke hit from the racquet side of the body.

Front Court: That section of the court in front of the service line.

Front Wall Kill: A kill shot that hits the front wall straight on and rebounds toward the back wall without touching a side wall.

Garbage Serve: A serve hit between the speed of a drive and a lob serve that bounces between the shoulder and waist to the receiver. The serve gives an illusion of a mis-hit serve.

Handout: Change of serves in double.

High-Z Serve: A serve that strikes high off the front wall (near the ceiling) and follows a "Z" pattern across the court.

Hinder: Any situation that prevents an opponent from having a fair shot at hitting the ball during a rally. Hinders include avoidable and dead-ball hinders.

Hyperthermia: Elevated body temperature.

Kill Shot: Any ball that strikes the front wall hard and low so the rebound with the floor occurs almost simultaneously with the wall. A winning offensive shot.

Lob: A defensive shot, hit along a side wall so it follows a path high over center court and falls with little rebound into a back corner. This ball may touch a side wall close to the back corner.

Long: A serve that strikes the back wall on the fly. A fault.

Match: The culmination of a competition with the winner usually winning two of three games. The first two games are played to 15 points; the third game, if required, is played to 11 points.

Mid-Court: The area between the service and short line and the two side walls.

Non-Thinking Strategy: Following a defensive reactive strategy with few decisions to make.

Offensive Shot: The attempt to win a point outright by virtue of the skill with which the shot is hit.

On Edge: The position of the racquet face when it is perpendicular to the floor.

Open Face: Position of the racquet face on the ball when hitting the ball up (usually turned toward the ceiling).

Out Serve: Serves including non-front wall serve, touched serve, crotch serve, illegal hit, out-of-order serve, safety zone violation, or fake serve, all resulting in a loss of serve.

Overhead: Shots hit from above the shoulder position with an extended arm.

Overhead Kill: A kill shot hit off a ball positioned above the shoulder.

Over-the-Shoulder: A ball hit from a position directly over the shoulder.

Passing Shot: An offensive shot that literally goes past an opponent who is in the front-, mid-, or center-court positions.

Pinch Kill: A shot that strikes the side wall–front wall sequence and that is unreturnable because of the low position, high velocity of the shot. Also called a pinch shot.

Protective Eyewear: Safety glasses required for wear when entering a racquetball court.

Racquet Face: The portion of the racquet with which the ball is struck during play.

Rally: An alternating, continuous exchange of shots during the play of a point.

Receiver: Player who receives the serve.

Receiving Line: The line identified by the intermittent floor marks located five feet behind the short line. A player may not stand in front of the receiving line to receive a serve.

Roll Out: A perfect kill shot defined by the action of the ball striking the front wall and rolling on the floor with no bounce.

Run the Corner: A ball that rebounds to a back corner, hitting the side wall and back wall before striking the floor.

Safety Hinder: When an opponent stops play to avoid contact with the other player that could result in injury.

Safety Zone: The 5-foot area defined by the area between the back edge of the short line and the receiving line. During the process of the serve, the receiver must wait for the ball to either bounce or cross the short line before stepping into the safety zone to return the serve.

Screen: A blocking of the opponent's vision, preventing the opponent from seeing the ball.

Service Box: The 18-inch box at each end of the service area where, in doubles, the server's partner stands until a legal serve has been executed by crossing the short line.

Service Line: The line on the floor closest to the front wall. The front line of the service zone.

Service Return: The shot hit in response to the serve at the beginning of each point.

Service Zone: The area between the service line and the short line. The area of the court for the server to legally execute the serve.

Set: The ready position. The position that enables the receiver of a shot to turn or pivot to hit the ball.

Setup: An easy shot that should be converted into an easy scoring opportunity for the hitter.

Short: A served ball that touches the floor in front of or on the short line. A fault.

Short Line: The back line of the service zone positioned 20 feet from the front wall. For a serve to be legal it must rebound past this line.

Sideout: A loss of a serve to the opponent.

Skip Ball: A shot that hits the floor before reaching the front wall. Usually a skip close to the front wall is difficult to determine.

Tether: The safety strap attached to the racquet grip and secured around the racquet wrist area. Also called a thong.

Thinking Strategy: The act of taking advantage of an opponent through the use of intellect, court strategy, and skill.

Three-Wall Racquetball: An alternative playing surface and court configuration minus a back wall and ceiling. With adaptation, games of singles, doubles, and cut-throat are played just as on a regulation four-wall court.

Three-Wall Shot: A defensive shot that rebounds off three walls.

Volley: Striking the ball in mid-air from a rebound off the front wall before the ball touches the floor.

Wallpaper Shot: A ball that rebounds along a side wall, making a return extremely difficult.

Warm-Up: Exercise engaged in before play that helps to prepare the body for activity.

Western Grip: A grip that is used for a forehand stroke. It is similar to the grip used on a racquet when it is picked up off the floor.

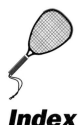

Index